HOLISTIC
STRENGTH TRAINING
FOR
TRIATHLON

Andrew Johnston
CHEK 3, HLC 3, USAT Level 1, CSCS, CPT

Former professional cyclist and current Ironman triathlete, leukemia survivor
and twice voted One of The 100 Best Trainers in America by Men's Journal

AuthorHouse™
1663 Liberty Drive
Bloomington, IN 47403
www.authorhouse.com
Phone: 1-800-839-8640

First published by AuthorHouse   2/21/2011

ISBN: 978-1-4567-2403-0 (sc)
ISBN: 978-1-4567-2404-7 (e)
ISBN: 978-1-4567-2405-4 (hc)

Library of Congress Control Number: 2010919579

Printed in the United States of America

TABLE OF CONTENTS

FOREWORD

The triathlete's body is subjected to a great deal of stress in each workout. Following the exercise protocols found in *Holistic Strength Training for Triathlon* will allow you to stay physically sound, recover well, and race fast. I highly recommend this work for triathletes who race at any distance.

As I read Andrew Johnston's book, I found myself repeatedly agreeing with his ways of preparing an athlete for serious training. After all, that's what flexibility, stability, and strength are—the building blocks for quality workouts. When these essentials are optimized with an increased emphasis early in your periodization plan, you will train well. Neglect these skills, however, and your risk of injury increases while your performance declines. The chapters of this guide are filled with vital information about the optimal preparation for (and, thus, optimal performance in) the sport of triathlon.

In *Holistic Strength Training for Triathlon*, Andrew Johnston has greatly expanded on topics I devoted only a few pages to in *The Triathlete's Training Bible*. He has not only dissected the subject of strength training for endurance sports, but he has also greatly refined the methodology. This makes his book a great resource to use in conjunction with *The Triathlete's Training Bible.*

Andrew's credentials for writing this book are excellent. He is a master coach with a wealth of athletic experience and sport science knowledge. All of this comes together very nicely on the pages of his text. *Holistic Strength Training for Triathlon* belongs on the shelf of any triathlete seeking a lifetime of healthy training and successful racing.

—Joe Friel

Joe Friel is one of the premier endurance coaches in the world with a client list that includes foreign and national champions, World Championship competitors, and even an Olympian. He is the author of ten books on training for endurance athletes including the popular and best-selling TrainingBible book series. He holds a masters degree in exercise science, is a USA Triathlon and USA Cycling certified Elite-level coach, and is a founder and past Chairman of the USA Triathlon National Coaching Commission.

ACKNOWLEDGMENTS

I will forever be indebted to Paul Chek. He is my teacher who became my mentor. And he is my mentor who I'm honored to say has become my friend. The education I have received during his four-year program, or even just four minutes in his presence, is forever life-changing. And as a CHEK Practitioner, I try to pay it forward, sharing his teachings with my family, my clients, or anyone within earshot (or even on Facebook). Any concept about which I write in this book that is not referenced can be directly or indirectly attributed to him. He was, unknowingly perhaps, my co-author.

There are many others whom I want to gratefully acknowledge here: Victoria Gammino for unpaid copy edits and (sometimes) brutal honesty on the text—I still owe you a dinner; Anna Branscome for *paid* copy edits which she subsequently donated to the Leukemia and Lymphoma Society in honor of her own mentor; Edward Wallace for designing the covers and layout of this book and being patient with me during the process; Rad Slough of Urban Body Fitness for allowing me to use his facility for the pictures of machines; Jennifer Schwartz for taking those pictures as well as the hundreds of shots we took in my studio—making me remotely photogenic takes incredible talent; Mary Campbell for the illustrations; Jennifer Wheelock for introducing me to Mary and Jill Joyner for connecting me with Anna; Berlin Berry for posing in a couple of the pictures with me—he's the taller one in the shots; Linda Burns, Nina Guzzetta, Bruce Johnston, Michael King, Dave Sierveld, Kathrine Tan, and Heather Weisenborn for reading my early drafts and responding with constructive criticism; and all of my clients whom I asked to read a sentence or look at a cover possibility—don't expect that much rest between sets always.

I'd also like to thank professional triathletes Blake Becker, Lewis Elliot, Heather Gollnick, and Caitlin Snow for taking time out of their busy schedules (and training for Kona) to read my manuscript and give me feedback. And special recognition goes to Joe Friel, author of *The Triathlete's Training Bible* and several other works, including the Foreword of this book. He was the first true expert in the field of training for endurance sports to read this book. And that he thought enough of my work to contribute to the project meant more to me than I can ever articulate—it's something I could never have imagined when I first read *The Cyclist's Training Bible* as an aspiring bike racer in college.

Additionally, I want to acknowledge my extended family. This includes the thousands of people who participate in Team in Training events worldwide as well as my brothers and sisters who fight alongside me in this war on cancer.

And the final thank you is reserved for my wife and son—Diana and Declan. Diana believed in my dreams, including the one which saw me living happily ever after with her. And Declan was patient while Daddy wrote this book. I've finished it now. Let's play, buddy.

INTRODUCTION

The body knows nothing of muscles, only movement. During the constant adaptive changes that must take place in order to preserve our equilibrium while moving, the body is constantly activating an array of muscles in patterns of coordination in which muscles lose their identity.

—Karl Bobath, MD

I never said thank you.

My first race after being diagnosed was the St. Anthony's Triathlon down in St. Pete, Florida. Racing was so much harder than I remembered, yet so much... I don't know... more. I can't tell you what it meant to be competing again. To have an actual line to cross to tell you that you've made it. I ran across the finish and fell into my wife's arms and we cried together, me hiding my face in her neck. I don't know if it was happiness or sadness or relief or what. It was probably just the fatigue from the race. And the deep, raw tiredness from emotions that can only be described as... alive!

And I was truly alive. I ended up placing in my age group and regret to this day that I didn't say something at the awards ceremony when they called my name. St. Anthony's is a big Team in Training event and the efforts of everyone involved in that organization raised over two million dollars that day for the Leukemia and Lymphoma Society. I should have said thank you; but really I was just too scared. I don't like talking in front of people. I don't really shine in the limelight. But all of those people deserved to know that this Team in Training thing really works.

This book is for them.

I've wanted to write this book for years. But I needed my opening line. I had to find my muse before I could make something of all the information I have: as a twenty-year veteran of cycling, as a professional cyclist in both the US and abroad from 1994-1998; as a multiple All-American triathlete, a Hawaii Ironman, and a cycling/triathlon coach for many seasons; as a personal trainer for over ten years, a Certified Strength and Conditioning Specialist since 2000, a Corrective Holistic Exercise Kinesiologist since 2001, and, most recently, as a leukemia survivor since August of 2004.

This book is my thank you.

If there's one thing cancer did for me, it gave me time. Funny to think that—that a disease which could so callously steal a person's years away would give me anything in return. But it has. It's given me a chance to work in instead of working out. It's allowed me to realize that the only time we truly have is Now. And now I'm going to take the advice of one of my college professors and write what I know.

I know triathlon. I'm familiar with the figures—ones which show that, in a five-year period, 90% of triathletes suffer an injury which results in the cessation of training. That's well above the average for athletes engaged in other endurance sports. Guess this kind of blows that cross-training argument out of the water. After all, aren't triathletes, by definition, cross training two-thirds of the time? True. But all this really means is that triathletes, of whom more than half are relatively inexperienced, have to navigate blindly the orthopedic demands of three sports instead of one.

People need to realize that exercise is powerful medicine. If you take the wrong drug, you're not going to get any better. Yet people are getting their prescription from their subscription! Triathletes, desperate for that competitive edge, are flipping through the pages of the latest multisport rag for some secret shortcut to the finish. Yet most of this information is general at best. Even the books specifically devoted to triathlon training usually have no more than an abbreviated chapter on weight training, with antiquated programs whose influences from the world of body building are plain to see. As two dimensional as the page it's written on, the program does little to prepare a person for the three-dimensional demands which triathlon places on the body.

It's time to take the strength-training program off the page, out of the gym, and into the competitive arena. How can you swim, bike, and run onto the podium if you can't even get to the starting line in one piece? Woody Allen said that 80% of success is just showing up. Yet apparently only one out of every ten triathletes can do this with a clean bill of health. Their preparation is lacking. One wouldn't just go out and play football with three-hundred-pound linemen without spending some structured time in the gym. But at the word "GO!" triathletes will try to tackle 6.2 miles in a fatigued state with impact forces during the course of the run amounting to well over five thousand times their own body weight! To stay healthy, the triathlete must be strong.

This book will show them how.

THE IMPORTANCE OF STRETCHING AND FLEXIBILITY

CHAPTER 1:

WHY START WITH STRETCHING?

If restored function and/or improved performance is the goal, a designed exercise program must first restore flexibility and stability to the working joints and balance the neuromuscular system. Next, strength is restored followed by re-establishing power output.

—Paul Chek

Flexibility before **Stability** before **Strength** before **Power**.

This is the functional progression which must be followed in any conditioning program. Breaking this chain will inevitably result in a broken athlete. Just like building a house, the foundation on which you build the body is critical to its future development and potential to weather any structural demands. While the house built outside the San Francisco area may never have to survive an earthquake, as athletes we *all* have to possess the specific attributes essential for successful completion of our next event or even our next workout. The physical skills to which I refer are listed by Tudor Bompa in his book *Theory and Methodology of Strength Training.* They are:

Agility
Balance
Coordination
Endurance
Power
Strength
Flexibility

Tudor calls these skills biomotor abilities. Bio = life; and motor = movement. Many of you reading this would argue that triathlon is life, and the rest is just details. So let's see how each of these qualities is necessary for us to swim, bike, and run.

Agility is the ability to move and change direction and position of the body quickly and effectively while under control. For the majority of us, it's the biomotor

17

ability of least importance to triathlon. In fact, some would say that the reason many of us were drawn to this sport in the first place is we have a distinct lack of the agility necessary for success in other sports. But, in truth, the ability to move quickly is essential for triathlon success. While we may not have to perform like dancers or martial artists, who hasn't looked at some elite runners in awe as they run with what could only be described as grace? As a professional cyclist, I was told to "dance on the pedals" when climbing a hill. And certainly a prerequisite of controlling the position of your body during a choppy open-water swim is agility.

Balance is another skill triathletes must master. Heck, juggling three different sports, a full-time job, the occasional shower, hectic family life, and some sense of mental and emotional stability is proof enough the multisport athlete must be practiced in the art of balance. From a physical standpoint, this biomotor ability helps us keep the rubber side down when on the bike. Balance in the water helps us swim with less drag. And running, which is essentially changing support from one leg to the other, is a practice in balance as we continually right ourselves over our feet.

Coordination refers to the ability to perform movements of various degrees of difficulty very quickly and with efficiency and accuracy. Quickness and efficiency during a triathlon will not only bring you across the finish line with a better time; coordinated movements will minimize the risk of injury as you swim, bike, and run. To maintain orthopedic integrity throughout a competitive career, the triathlete must possess a high level of coordination among all three disciplines.

Endurance is the most obvious of the biomotor abilities the triathlete must have. Also known as stamina, endurance is the ability to perform work of a given intensity over a specified time period or distance. Whether it's a sprint or an Ironman, triathletes must be able to resist fatigue. Simply logging miles in the pool, in the saddle, or on your legs is one way to build endurance. But we all have a limited amount of time we can allot to training before life gets in the way. So maximizing this skill at the same time others are developed is the hallmark of the intelligent multisport athlete.

Power is the ability to apply force quickly. All movements require some degree of power, and the three activities which make up a triathlon are no exception. A combination of strength and speed, power is yet another determinant of who crosses the line first in a triathlon. Among hypothetical comparisons or real-life examples, all things being equal, the more powerful triathlete will always have a higher placing than the other. For a more comprehensive discussion, refer to the third section of this book so you can enhance your understanding of this critical biomotor ability. After all, knowledge is power.

Strength is what this book is all about. Defined as the state, quality, or property of being physically or mentally strong, any triathlete will vouch for the importance of a strong mind. The debate over strength training for physical performance, however, is one which has sparked passionate if not misguided discussion among swimmers, cyclists, and runners for years. The third section of this book is devoted to a detailed discussion of how this biomotor ability is essential for the triathlete, and should convince even the most rabid of strength training's detractors to spend some time in the weight room. But while the chapter titled "Nutrition and Lifestyle Considerations for Optimal Performance" later in the book will address the principle of thinking, a detailed discussion of mental strength and psychological training is beyond the scope of this writing.

Flexibility is the ability to adapt to changes in position or alignment, allowing us to perform joint actions through a wide range of motion. Often used interchangeably with mobility, which can be defined as the ability to move freely, these two concepts are the heart of this chapter. They're also the heart of the biomotor abilities above. Think about it—how agile can you be if your muscles are stiff? Have you ever cramped during a triathlon? Your ability to move or change direction quickly was instantly curtailed. In fact, if you weren't stopped dead in your tracks, you probably looked like the Tin Man trying to jog a couple of days after hanging out in the rain all night. Being too tight also affects your balance. Pulled out of ideal alignment by tonic musculature, you are literally over-committed in one direction. Coordination will suffer, too, as a lack of mobility must be compensated for elsewhere in the kinetic chain, often resulting in inefficiency and injury. With altered length/tension relationships, the triathlete must now work harder to perform a given movement which adversely affects endurance. Muscles positioned outside of their optimal strength curve will not only be weaker but, since strength is a component of power, a final injustice to the inflexible triathlete is that these last two biomotor abilities will never reach their full potential—much like this triathlete and his placement in the overall field.

CHAPTER 2:

PHASIC vs. TONIC MUSCULATURE

To stretch or not to stretch? That is **not** the question. Not really. Though there are numerous studies debating the merits of stretching, the ones which find no benefit to the athlete are typically flawed. The authors researching the efficacy of stretching inevitably apply a general stretching protocol to the subjects in their study with a one-size-fits-all mentality. But different activities cause different responses in different muscles. This is simple to understand when one considers that not all muscles are created equal. For the purpose of this discussion, I will focus on the difference between **Phasic** muscles and **Tonic** muscles.

Phasic Muscles *are composed of at least 51%* ***fast-twitch*** *muscle fibers. These are powerful muscles, but they fatigue more easily than do tonic muscles. Kind of a shame, too, as these muscles are primarily responsible for movement. The gluteals are good examples of phasic muscles.*

Tonic Muscles *are* ***slow-twitch*** *dominant, composed of at least 51% slow-twitch muscle fibers. As such, they are highly resistant to fatigue and have a greater propensity for work. The iliopsoas is an example of a tonic muscle group.*

The table below categorizes some of the more common muscles as either Phasic or Tonic:

Properties of Tonic and Phasic Musculature

Predominantly Tonic Muscles	Predominantly Phasic Muscles
Prone to Hyperactivity	Prone to Inhibition
Function	
Posture	Movement
Susceptibility to Fatigue	
Late	Early
Reaction to Faulty Loading	
Shortening	Weakening
Shoulder Girdle – Arm	
Pectoralis Minor Levator Scapulae Trapezius (upper) Biceps Brachii Scalenes Subscapularis Sternocleidomastoids Masticatory Forearm Flexors	Rhomboids Trapezius (middle) Trapezius (lower) Triceps Brachii Deep Neck Flexors Forearm Extensors Supraspinatus Infraspinatus Serratus lateralis Deltoid
Trunk	
Lumbar and Cervical Erectors Quadratus Lumborum	Thoracic Erectors Rectus Abdominis
Pelvis – Thigh	
Hamstrings Iliopsoas Rectus Femoris Thigh Adductors Piriformis Tensor Fasciae Latae	Vastus Lateralis Vastus Medialis Gluteal Muscles
Lower Leg – Foot	
Gastrocnemius Soleus	Anterior Tibialis Peroneals Extensors of the toes

One of the major differences between phasic and tonic muscles that is of particular interest to triathletes is how these muscles respond to faulty loading. Loading is the resistance which the muscles of the body must overcome. In the gym, it may be a dumbbell. In life, it's gravity. Thus, even if the only weight room you've ever spent time in is the wait room at your doctor's office, it's fair to say we all experience loading in our lives. Faulty loading can take the form of under-use, misuse, or disuse. But as triathletes, who swim, bike, and run for up to seventeen hours all in the same day, the form of faulty loading we are typically concerned with is overuse.

Tonic muscles respond to faulty loading by shortening and tightening. With a lower threshold for stimulation, tonic muscles need very little encouragement to turn on. This can, and often does, result in hyperactivity of a tonic muscle, limiting the motion at the joint(s) over which that muscle crosses. As mentioned in the preceding chapter, this lack of flexibility (or more specifically, this lack of mobility) results in all the biomotor abilities being adversely affected.

Phasic musculature does the exact opposite. It tends to lengthen and weaken in relation to its relative antagonist(s) or opposing muscle (group). The problem is then magnified by the fact that muscles which are short and tight will hold their antagonists in a lengthened position. This can lead to what is commonly termed **stretch weakness**. Stretch weakness is defined by Florence Kendall in her book entitled *Muscles: Testing and Function with Posture and Pain* as

23

> *weakness that results from muscles remaining in an elongated condition,*
>
> *however slight, beyond the neutral physiological rest position, but not*
>
> *beyond the normal range of muscle length.*

She goes on to say that "the concept relates to the *duration* of the faulty alignment rather than the *severity* of it" (italics mine). So is it any surprise that the aspiring triathlete, who may spend up to *seven hours at a time* hunched over the bike with a rounded back, has increased thoracic **kyphosis** and can't stand up straight? Brick that with a swim where the pectorals and medial shoulder rotators get overworked during the course of an hour-and-a-half-pool session, and the source of the typical triathlete's faulty posture becomes clear. Now the lengthened muscles of the thoracic spine are being pulled by the tight muscles of the chest, shoulders, and lats. This results in even more thoracic kyphosis.

Maybe you should just run, you're thinking. Well, the increased lumbar curvature created by the tight, overworked quads and hip flexors of the average runner causes a compensation in the thoracic spine leading to… say it with me… *increased thoracic kyphosis.* So much for the benefits of cross training, right? Instead of one source for our orthopedic and postural aberrations, we triathletes have three. I guess we're just S.O.L.

But no, we're not out of luck. We just can't rely on dumb luck when it comes to our stretching program. We can't just do random stretches for every part of the body and expect our sport-specific muscle imbalances to be addressed. We need a specific course of stretching which actively targets the muscles we abuse when we swim, bike, and run.

The question then isn't if to stretch, but when to stretch and how? If you perform stretches for every part of the body, you haven't done anything to alleviate the muscle imbalance caused by your triathlon training. The tight muscles are still tighter than the loose ones. Your body is still out of alignment. And a body that's not properly aligned moves and functions less efficiently, increasing its susceptibility to fatigue and, ultimately, to injury.

The bicycle wheel is a common analogy which effectively represents this idea. Ideally, thirty-two spokes running from the rim to the hub are tensioned appropriately to keep the wheel spinning true. Logging a lot of miles on the bike, especially under harsh road conditions with bumps or potholes, can lead to a wheel which wobbles as certain spokes get tighter while others become looser. Each imperfection in the road leads to the wheel wobbling worse and worse.

During college, I worked in a bike shop in St. Petersburg, Florida. Some Mondays, guys would come in with their wheels after crashing at the weekend's bike race to see if the wheels were salvageable. The head mechanic, a guy named Ray who worked wonders with the spoke wrench, would stick the wheel in the truing stand and spin it. The arms of the stand would tell him which spokes were in need of tightening and which should be loosened. He'd keep fine tuning the calibration of the stand—tightening a spoke half a turn here, loosening another with a quarter turn—until the wheel ran as straight and true as the day the cyclist bought it.

Some wheels, and some cyclists, weren't so lucky. One day a guy in shredded Lycra limped into the shop carrying his mountain bike. He'd gone down pretty hard on a training ride and his front wheel was so out of true he'd had to walk the bike to the store. The guy asked us if we could fix it enough for him to ride it home. Not much for words, Ray took the wheel from the guy, went behind the counter, and held it up at eye level as if he were reading which spokes needed attention. Suddenly, and with force which could be heard over the Chili Peppers playing on the shop's stereo, he slammed the wheel down hub-first again and again. After a few seconds, he paused, repositioned the wheel in his hands like a guy making a pizza, and slammed it down on the counter a few more times. Finally, he stopped banging the wheel and gave it back to the cyclist, who looked a bit more abused than when he'd come in. But his face changed as he spun the wheel. It still wobbled. But if he could endure a jerky ride, the wheel looked like it just might get him home.

Throughout the body, ideal length-tension relationships exist which, when altered by chronic shortening or lengthening of certain muscles, result in faulty joint kinematics. It's a matter of physics. Forces generated by movement or loading cannot be adequately dissipated in a joint which has moved away from its instantaneous axis of rotation. The resulting premature degradation of the joint itself inevitably hastens the demise of the triathlete's competitive career. But if you stretch the right muscles at the right time and in the right way, just like a wheel in a truing stand, your chances of maintaining your orthopedic integrity increase exponentially. And though I can't promise you that you won't ever have to walk your *bike* home, with correct stretching you should never have to limp your *body* home.

CHAPTER 3:
WHICH, WHEN, AND HOW?

One must determine the overall objectives of treatment based on whether stability or mobility is the desired outcome for optimal function. Joint structures are so designed that along with greater mobility there is less stability, and along with greater stability there is less mobility.

—Florence Kendall

Which muscles are the ones you need to stretch? Easy: the short tight ones. Simply put, if it's not tight, then don't stretch it! Don't overthink this one. It doesn't have to be rocket science. If you perform any of the stretches listed, and the muscle doesn't feel tight, then you don't need to do that particular stretch. The muscle groups the typical triathlete often needs to focus on are:

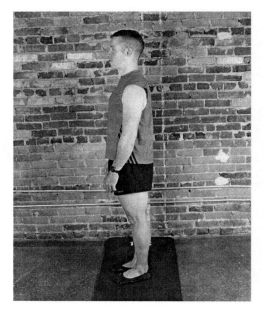 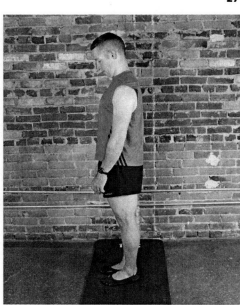

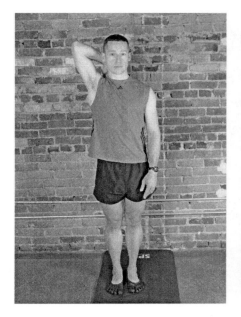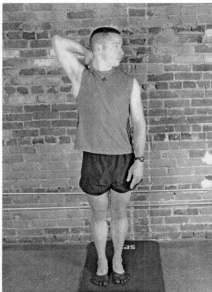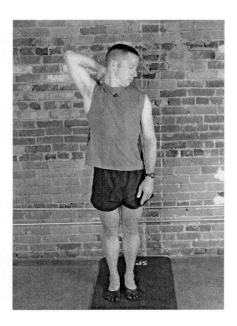

LEVATOR SCAPULAE

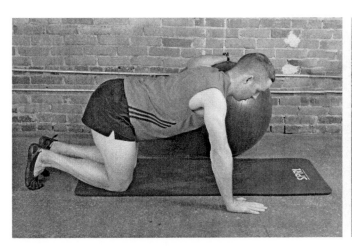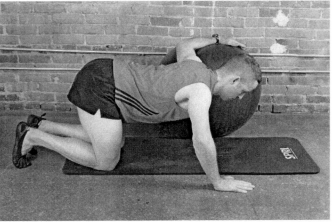

PECTORALIS

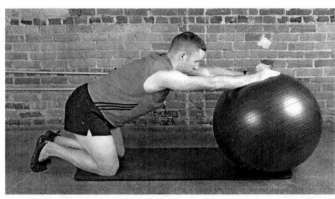

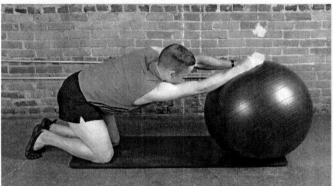

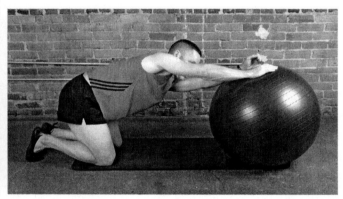

LATISSIMUS DORSI

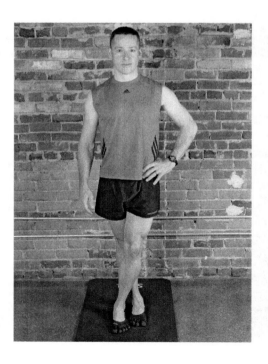

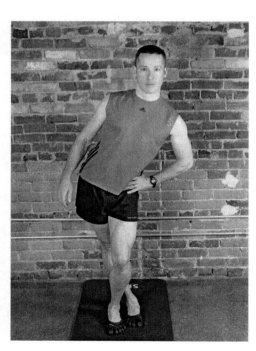

ILIOTIBIAL BAND

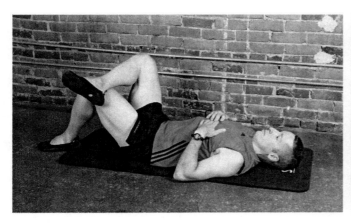 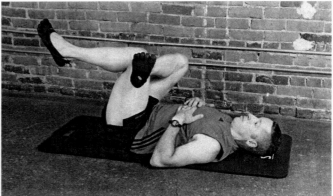

EXTERNAL HIP ROTATORS

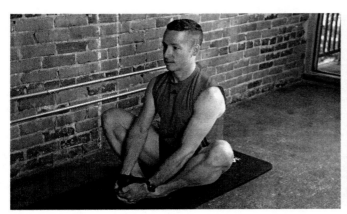 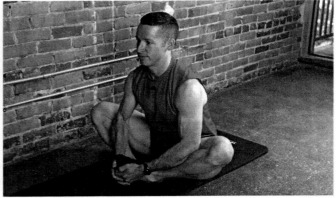

INTERNAL HIP ROTATORS

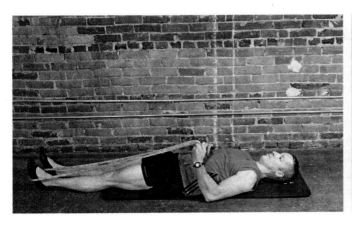 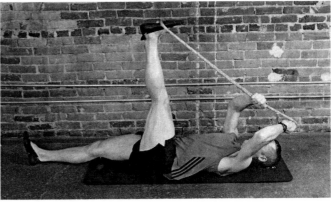

HAMSTRINGS

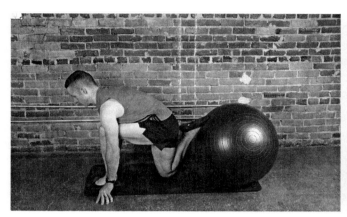

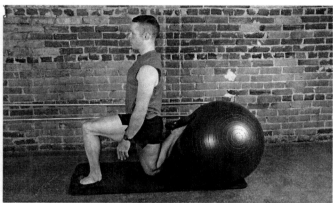

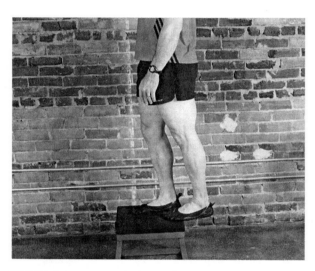

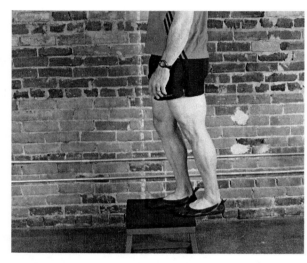

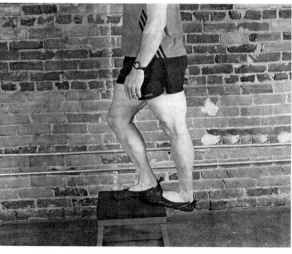

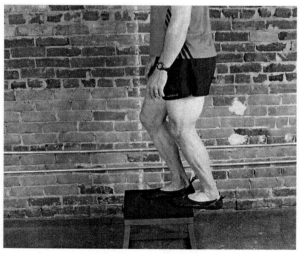

GASTROCNEMIUS

SOLEUS

When to stretch is a bit more complex. A study in the Journal of Applied Physiology found that prolonged (thirty seconds or longer) or **static stretching** decreases strength for up to one hour in the specific muscle stretched due to altered activation and contractile force.

So what are you thinking now when you see your competitors bending down to touch their toes and holding that position for the last few minutes before an event? You should be licking your chops! With every second some guy in your age group holds a particular stretch, the likelihood of you taking home the hardware he thought was rightfully his increases. As researchers Nelson, Kokkonen, and Arnall explain it,

> *the stretching regimen placed a proportion of the motor units into a fatiguelike state prior to the initiation of the (event). Placing specific motor units into a fatiguelike state would decrease the pool of motor units available for activation, and this loss of motor units from the pool of available motor units could hasten the fatigue and lead to a decrease in performance.*

All these stretching zealots have it backwards. Static stretching works through a process called autogenic inhibition whereby the Golgi tendon organ is stimulated and an inhibitory effect on the muscle spindle is created. And it is quite effective in elongating the soft tissue of the body. But based on the above research, static stretching is best done **after** exercise to help "re-set" the muscles used during the activity to their ideal resting length, further ingraining the proper motor engram—the memorized motor pattern used to perform a specific movement or skill—into the neuromuscular system. This will help implant in the muscle's memory the range of motion necessary for the health and performance of the triathlete.

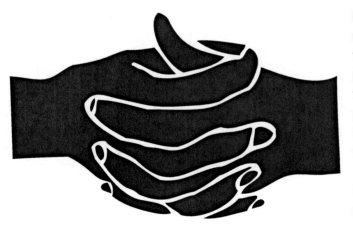

Did you think your brain had a monopoly on memory? Hardly! In fact, if you'll put your hands together and interlace your fingers like you're praying, you'll see what I'm talking about. I know that most triathlons are held on Sunday, and you probably haven't stepped foot in a church in years. But you still know how to pray. So put your hands together like I instructed.

Now, open your hands and interlace your fingers so that the opposite thumb is on top. Feels wrong, doesn't it? And to your body it is. This is not the motor engram your body has been programmed with for years. This is not what your body *remembers* as correct.

And I know I'm going to get some nasty feedback for these next couple of lines, but muscle memory* is the reason why you have to visit your chiropractor's clinic once a week or more. Many chiropractors try to fix subluxations—a joint which is out of place and causing discomfort or dysfunction—by adjusting the bones. But bones don't have memory. So unless your doctor also addresses the muscles, as soon as you get off the treatment table your body is pulling you back into the exact same faulty position which brought you into the clinic in the first place.

Thus, every time you take your body through a workout, whether it is weights or swimming or Sweating to the Oldies with Richard Simmons, the muscles involved in the activity are "taught" that their ideal resting length is short and tight, if you fail to stretch them afterwards. This is the position which they will remember. Therefore, you must stretch the muscles after your workout so that they "learn" their proper length-tension relationships. Failure to do so eventually has catastrophic results. Muscles become tighter and tighter while the body gets thrown more and more out of balance. Perform a movement with a body which is out of balance, and the nervous system must figure out a way to compensate. And all too often these compensations result in faulty movement patterns which are inefficient and dangerous to the integrity of the joints and all their accompanying structures. As Kendall states:

> When there is normal movement in joints, wear and tear on joint surfaces tends to be distributed; however, if there is limitation of range, the wear will take place only on the joint surfaces that represent the arc of use. If the part that is restricted by muscle tightness is protected against any movement that may cause strain, other parts that must compensate for such restrictions will suffer the strain instead.

33

*More accurately, there is no such thing as muscle memory. Rather it is the brain and spinal cord which create the motor engram of a specific movement or position.

CHAPTER 4:

STRETCHES? WE DON'T NEED NO STINKING STRETCHES!

Perhaps you didn't know the exact mechanism by which stretching helps reduce the possibility of injury. Maybe you never bought into the idea that taking your muscles to the point of tension and holding them there for thirty to sixty seconds would make you a better triathlete. After all, you have a friend who's as flexible as Gumby on muscle relaxers. She does twenty minutes of stretching before brushing her teeth, for crying out loud. Yet, she's constantly injured. That's the only research you ever needed to convince you that stretching was a waste of time.

Aaron Mattes, author of *Active Isolated Stretching*, cites the following benefits of an optimal flexibility program:

- Athletes reach peak performance sooner and sustain it longer.

- Muscles respond more quickly and powerfully.

- Performance is improved with reduced chance of injury.

- Muscle stiffness is reduced as excess lactic acid buildup is removed. Reduction in metabolic wastes allows muscles to rejuvenate more quickly after intense workouts or athletic events.

- Athletes recuperate more quickly. Healing of injuries is faster and stronger without the loss of power due to the development of transverse fibrosis.

- There is a reduction in spasms, splinting, and tension as a result of ischemia.

- Athletes increase their career span and level of performance.

And now that you know that static stretching needs to be performed **after** your training, you can maximize the above benefits without risk of sacrificing your athletic performance. However, since the body always gravitates toward a position of strength, failure to stretch **before** a workout only ingrains any postural aberrations more deeply into your neuromuscular system as you literally strengthen yourself in a position of poor posture.

So what's the answer?

Instead of holding your stretches and inhibiting the very muscles with which you need to compete, you should use **dynamic stretching** before a workout or race. This protocol employs controlled, constant movement into and out of a stretch position until the athlete begins to feel limber. Instead of turning the muscles off, dynamic stretching actually excites the neuromuscular system, and prepares it for the activity to come. The triathlete should target all the major muscle groups used in triathlon, remembering to move neither too quickly and bounce (i.e., ballistic stretching) or to hold an end position for longer than two seconds (i.e., static stretching).

There is, of course, one exception to this rule, too. Musculature which you have identified as tonic (either through the help of a CHEK practitioner (https://www.chekconnect.com/), via the tests in this book, or maybe through your own experience) needs to be addressed prior to exercise with good old static stretching. This will help calm the tonic muscles. And why, you ask, would you want to sedate any muscle prior to competition or training? Well, if you have a group of muscles which are easily facilitated and have a tendency to do the work of their functional antagonists, what do you think is the inevitable outcome of such a scenario?

Let's play this out. Through a process called **reciprocal inhibition**, a muscle will relax to accommodate the contraction of its opposing muscle. For example, as the quadricep contracts to extend the leg during the push phase of the pedal stroke, the hamstring relaxes and moves into an elongated position. Yet with an overly excited, tonic muscle, some of the neural drive to the **prime mover** is "stolen" to maintain its chronic level of excitation. In the pedaling scenario above, if the hamstrings are constantly turned on, then the neural drive which should be reserved for quadricep contraction is often robbed. This can result in decreased force production by the affected muscle, forcing the **_synergists_** of this muscle to "pick up the slack." Unable to maintain optimal force production during a task they were really not designed to handle, the synergists become fatigued and the eventual degradation of a specific movement pattern ultimately results in injury.

The late Vladimir Janda, one of the premier manual therapists in the rehabilitative world, would have probably agreed that the psoas is the perfect tonic muscle to illustrate this phenomenon. When overly excited, the psoas causes its antagonist, the gluteus maximus, to become inhibited. In addition to their contribution to **frontal plane** stability, the gluteals are active in the propulsive phase of running as they push downwards and backwards in concert with the hamstrings. But if the gluteals are inhibited because their neural energy is being stolen by the psoas, the hamstrings now have to create hip extension on their own. This not only results in a less powerful push-off, but now the hamstrings are getting overworked.

But there's more. Look at the table above, and you'll see that the hamstrings are tonic muscles and, thus, respond to faulty loading by shortening and tightening. Antagonistic to the quadriceps, which are also involved in providing forward thrust in running, tight hamstrings can limit the maintenance of an efficient stride as they rob the quadriceps, specifically the vastus medialis and lateralis, of their neural impulse. Then the snowball gets bigger. Or the whirlpool spins faster. Or the dominoes keep falling. Use whatever analogy seems most appropriate: The eventual outcome is the same. The entire **kinetic chain** is drawn into a quagmire of dysfunction which steadily pulls the athlete down into injury. And unless you want to follow this hypothetical athlete in his decline, you'd better turn off those tonic muscles.

IN SUMMARY:

Pre-Workout/Race
Dynamic stretching
Static stretching of any *tonic* musculature

Post-Workout/Race
Static stretching

37

CHAPTER 5:
SELF-MYOFASCIAL RELEASE

In addition to muscles, tendons, and ligaments, the body's soft tissue is composed of a fourth important substance called **fascia**. Much like the wrapping of a mummy, fascia is a dense, subcutaneous connective tissue which extends from head to toe without interruption. In a healthy state it stretches and moves without restriction, effectively connecting your entire body, from your toenails to your eyelashes. Therefore, distortion of the fascial system through any trauma (i.e., overuse or faulty posture or even emotional turmoil) can interfere with the proper functioning of every bone, muscle, or nerve in the body. Mattes explains,

The fascial network of the body responds effectively to external forces such as trauma, overuse syndromes, and poor physical mechanics. In these circumstances, external forces affect the body over short and long periods of time, challenging the fascia to maintain functional integrity and homeostasis. External environmental trauma alters both the contractile force of the collagenous fibers and the thixotropic hardening of the ground substance. This causes a disruption in the movement of the muscular tissue, neurological impulses, channeling of blood and lymphatic fluids, hydration, oxygenation, and nutritional homeostasis. Restoring the physiological process continually require adaptations within the three-dimensional fascial fibrous matrix primarily on the subcutaneous fascial plane. Myofascial motion facilitates hydration, oxygenation, and removal of toxins and promotes healing.

Stretching is one of the easiest ways for the triathlete to achieve this myofascial motion. Yet Mattes warns that "only relaxed myofascial structures will allow themselves to be optimally stretched." In other words, stretch until the cows come home. But until you get any myofascial restrictions to release, you continue to "promote detrimental contractures, inflammation, lymphatic congestion, peripheral vascular obstruction, hypertension, and a host of other disease states." And, personally, I have a hard enough time remembering to take my helmet off before running out of T2 (like I did in my first *and* second duathlons) without having to worry about "peripheral vascular obstruction" or any of those other problems.

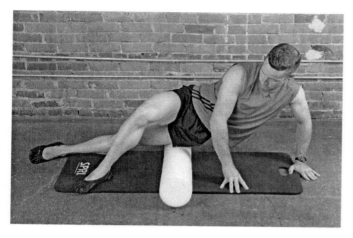

FOAM ROLLER

The most practical method to relax a specific myofascial structure is through the use of a foam roller. First the athlete rolls on the foam roller, trying to locate any knots or adhesions—the normally separate anatomical structures which have "glued" together through an ironic combination of neglect and overuse to form what is essentially an unhealthy band of scar tissue. You'll know you've found one when your body involuntarily tries to jump off the foam roller as you grimace in agony with cold beads of sweat running down your forehead. I suggest searching on your lateral thigh along the infamous I.T. band as demonstrated in the picture to the left. This should take all of about two nanoseconds for most triathletes before a "trigger point" is found. Then, using the weight of the body, apply tolerable pressure to the area for thirty seconds or more until the pain subsides.

This allows the bundled collagenous fibers of the adhesion to be realigned properly in the direction of the muscle fiber so that the fascia can relax. It also allows the triathlete to put in perspective what real pain is, making the discomfort endured during the course of any triathlon appear relatively minor in comparison. Once the adhesion relaxes, the athlete rolls on until he finds the next trouble spot and repeats the process.

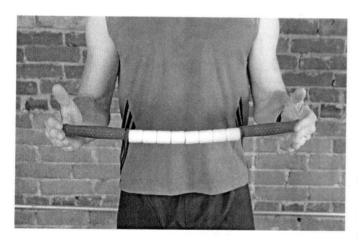

THE STICK

The Stick is another tool the triathlete can use to achieve myofascial release while more easily accommodating the limitations of a pre-race or pre-workout environment. Basically, it's a small, plastic device which looks much like a rolling pin. But you're not kneading dough—you're kneading out the knots and scar tissue in your muscles that have developed over the course of hundreds or even thousands of hours of training.

My first introduction to The Stick came in 1996 when Eric Gonstead, a chiropractor friend of mine, mailed me a care package in Spain, where I was based for the season. Eric was a really strong cyclist and former triathlete whose demanding class schedule, as well as an affinity for Guinness, took his athletic ambitions down a path a little less lofty than my own. He lived vicariously through me, taking a special interest in my cycling career and earning my trust both as a friend and as a doctor. So when he sent me The Stick, I immediately began to use it. What the heck? My teammates, who were from more conservative countries like Spain, France, Denmark, and Russia, found me and some of my American race rituals (like drinking enough water during a race) a bit strange anyway.

Then, in 2001, while working as performance coach at Velocity Sports Performance in Marietta, Georgia, I was instructed in the use of The Stick in a more formal setting. I was responsible for the training of various athletes, from football players to figure skaters. And one of my duties was taking them through a ten-minute "Stick protocol" before any of the athletes were allowed to continue with the demands of the more structured training programs. Velocity was at the cutting edge of training for sports. That the head coaches there, Loren Seagraves and John Crosby, thought enough of the benefits of The Stick to include it in the training of all their athletes impressed me. When the bobsledders they were training became the first team from the United States to ever medal in the Winter Olympics—with GOLD no less—I was a Stick convert!

And if I hadn't been a disciple of The Stick before, I soon became a zealot when I came across an article by Rex Reese about Lance Armstrong and his 2002 United States Postal Cycling Team. In it was an interview with the team chiropractor, Jeff Spencer, about his duties during the team's assault on the Tour de France. Jeff was taking around $60,000 worth of equipment overseas to keep the team healthy, everything from an Erchonia cold laser to a piece of equipment called the "H-Wave." Also included in his arsenal of treatment modalities, and "no less important than the most expensive equipment," he used was The Stick. Well, if it's good enough for Lance...

41

CHAPTER 6:
THE WARM UP

I've never tried to foam roll while in my car before a race, but I've worked with The Stick on several cold race mornings when the weather and my lack of foresight forced me to warm up in the confines of my back seat. One of those races was Powerman Alabama. It was late March in the South, so I hadn't even dreamed of packing arm warmers or tights or anything to help combat the sub-40° temps and wind which greeted me and the other thousand athletes on race morning. And I suck in the cold. I'm one of those guys who'll tear your legs off when it's 100° outside. Yet I suffer like a dog in the cold. Cold and wet and I get dropped like your bike box at the airport. Makes me wonder how I survived two racing seasons in Belgium.

A proper warm up should raise the temperature of the body by one or two degrees Celsius (1.4° to 2.8° Fahrenheit). According to *Stretching Scientifically: A Guide to Flexibility Training* by Tom Kurz, a good warm up will increase awareness, improve coordination, improve elasticity and contractibility of muscles, lubricate the working joints, as well as heighten the efficiency of the respiratory and cardiovascular systems. Additionally, dilation of the blood vessels will occur, resulting in improvement of the body's cooling efficiency. Activation of enzymes responsible for energy metabolism will also be increased. One final benefit will be higher levels of excitation in both the nervous and hormonal systems so that the body is primed for peak physical performance.

43

Well, without the right type of clothing, I wasn't going to go outside until the announcer called us to the line. I had a heater in the car. So I huddled in the passenger seat with my wife sweating buckets as I cranked the heat and took myself through an extended Stick session. Literally three minutes before the gun, I hopped out of the car and jogged to the start while doing some running drills. I knew it wasn't the ideal warm up. But I didn't have time to worry about it as I made it to the start line just as the announcer yelled "GO!"

If I had been able to do my normal warm up, it would have looked something like this:

Fifty strokes with The Stick on the calves, the hamstrings, the quads, the glutes, and lumbar erectors.

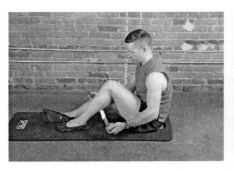 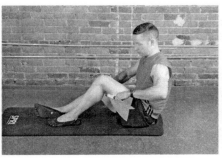 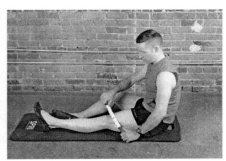

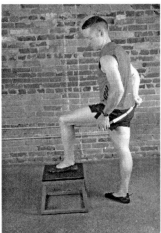 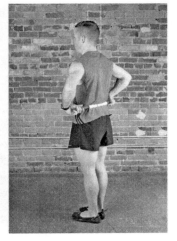

Walking for three to five minutes while gently rotating specific body parts in clockwise and counterclockwise motions to lubricate the joints with synovial fluid to help reduce the normal friction associated with movement:

wrists	**elbows**
shoulders	**waist**
hips	**knees**
ankles	

Dynamic stretching of all muscles used in the event plus specific movements including:

pectoralis major/minor

latissimus dorsi

external/internal hip rotators

quadriceps/hip flexors

hamstrings

gastroc/soleus

squats (see p.167)

lunges (see p.172)

Static stretching (if necessary) of any musculature which may be chronically tight or facilitated.

Gradually progress from a walk to a jog and then to a series of drills performed for ten meters or ten seconds:

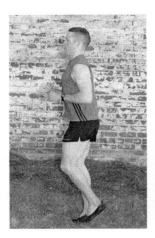 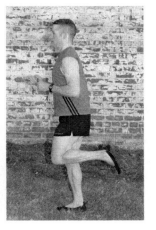

BUTT KICKS

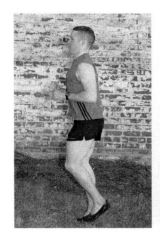 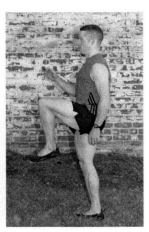

HIGH KNEES

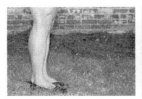 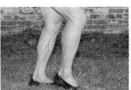 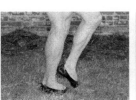 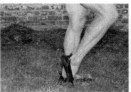 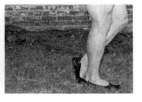

ANKLING

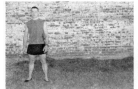 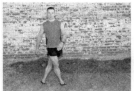 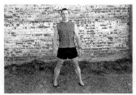 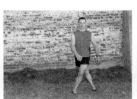 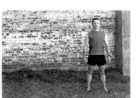

CARIOCA

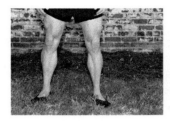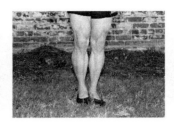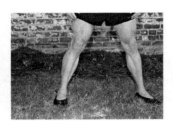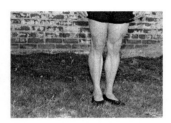

SIDE GLIDES

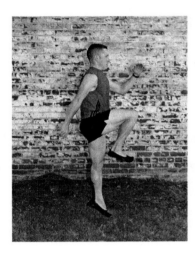

SKIPPING

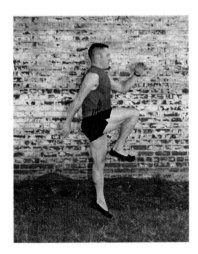

POWERSKIPS

To make sure my system was primed and ready to perform, I'd run several 50 to 100 meter sprints of increasing intensity with light jogging in between each effort. Then I'd camp out near the start line to ensure I was near the front when the gun sounded as I performed **flicks** with my arms and legs. This final aspect of my warm up would be sure to earn me some weird glances from anyone around me. When I'm doing these, I look like I'm flicking invisible flies off my hands and feet but in a rhythmic fashion. And that's actually a pretty good description of how to do them. And why do I do them? I'm sure you're not the first person to ask that during my pre-race ritual.

The physiological justification for doing them is to relax my muscles and decompress my joints, allowing my body to move freely and without energy-sapping compensations that could result in injury. In his book, *The Golf Biomechanic's Manual*, Paul Chek says these flicks restore non-physiological joint motion and uses the analogy of a bicycle headset to aid the reader's understanding. If you over-tighten this "joint" on your bike, the handlebars don't move easily and more force is required to turn it. Likewise, if excessive muscle tension and joint pressure restrict the motion of your body, it's going to be a bitch to get it to swim, bike, and run. Even if you still don't buy my explanation and think "flicks" are just a nervous habit for me, you have to admit: It's better than biting my nails...

THE CORE CONCEPTS OF STABILITY

CHAPTER 1:

MACHINE MAYHEM

Core is a hot word in the fitness industry these days. There are as many articles on developing "six-pack" abs as there seems to be stud triathletes competing for a Kona slot in your age group. But the core is much more than a washboard stomach.

The core consists of:

- The four abdominal muscles (external oblique, internal oblique, rectus abdominus, and transversus abdominus (TVA))

- The muscles of the spine including the Erector Spinae Group (iliocostalis, longissimus, and spinalis), the Transversospinalis Group (multifidi, rotatores, semispinalis), the latissimus dorsi, and the quadratus lumborum

- The thoracolumbar aponeurosis

- The hip musculature (adductors, gluteals, and iliopsoas)

- The muscles of the pelvic floor

- The diaphragm

49

In addition, the muscles of the cervical and thoracic spine contribute to the integrity of the core, and thus should be included in this discussion. The internal organs also constitute the core, but their inclusion goes beyond the scope of this writing.

Machine training causes what I like to call "core amnesia." Machines obviate the need for balance as you exert force. Typically, you are seated and forced into a position that does not accommodate your specific body type, on a big hunk of metal with a fixed axis of rotation. You could literally "exercise" through an earthquake measuring 7.5 on the Richter Scale—the machine is bolted to the floor, after all, so you don't even have to think about your core, much less worry about activating it. And if you don't use it, guess what—you lose it.

As world-renowned strength coach Charles Poliquin so eloquently says, "You can't fire a cannon from a canoe." Stability *must* precede force production. If you have lost the ability to activate your core properly, either from lack of use or from a faulty conditioning program, movements of the arms and the legs will not have a stable base from which to produce power. This is critical, as research from a 1999 book about spinal stabilization concluded that specific core musculature is activated thirty milliseconds before arm movements (i.e., swimming) and 110 milliseconds before leg movement (i.e., cycling or running). That is, if the core is functioning properly!

And if it's not? If you've been dutifully working out on machines and the musculature of your trunk can't remember where the on switch is? Well, without adequate core stability, an athlete is unable to provide the proper foundation necessary to apply force through the extremities. He can shoot his cannons. But his gym-built battleship physique gets pushed backwards. If he fires his cannons again, his bow might go under. Soon he'll be taking on water. Then it's only a matter of time until he sinks into injury.

Thomas Hanna, author of *Bodies in Revolt*, popularized the term "sensory-motor amnesia" in 1988 to describe the inability to activate a specific muscle due to a lack of sensory input to that muscle. Like I said above—if you don't use it, you lose it! And the last thing anyone needs, especially a triathlete, is a core with Alzheimer's. He goes on to say that "perhaps as many as fifty percent of the cases of chronic pain suffered by human beings are caused by sensory-motor amnesia (SMA)."

As triathletes, we're all familiar with pain. The test of a triathlon, though taken in the presence of others, is one which ultimately measures how far we're willing to push *ourselves*, how much discomfort we can endure. Yet as soon as we cross the finish line, the burning lungs and screaming muscles immediately begin to fade into memory.

Chronic pain is different. Unfortunately, though, far too many triathletes have found that chronic pain is their most reliable training partner, never missing a workout. Even on "good" days when the pain seems gone, it haunts our thoughts. We wonder if the next step or the next stroke will be the one which makes us realize that the pain is still there. And no matter how far we go or how fast we train, we can't seem to drop it. It's so damn frustrating! But if Thomas Hanna is correct, could half of us be pain free if we simply learned to activate specific muscles correctly? Are there simple steps we could take so that pain realizes that the invitation to train with us has been rescinded?

Well, as far as the core is concerned, we could get into a position which actually requires these muscles to work! With patience, I've been able to teach this critical position successfully to 100% of my clients. So if you'll read the following instructions carefully and practice with dutiful attention to form, in time, you, too, will master this movement.

First, I want you to stand up.

That's it.

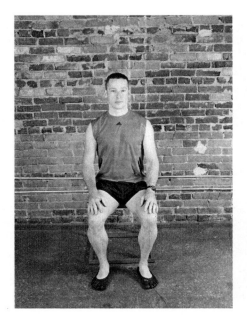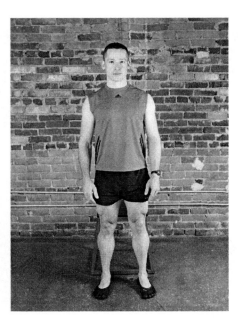

Can you believe it? *Just stand up!* Now your core is turned on. It wasn't that hard now, was it? Admittedly, you now have to do things you never had to do while working on a machine—like dealing with balance and gravity and engaging muscles which were turned off before. But the advantages to your lower back should make these sacrifices worth it. While people complaining of back pain are frequently told to sit down, doing so can actually be contraindicated. "Taking the load off" literally puts the load on. Lumbar disc pressures are 40% higher in a seated position than when standing. With poor posture, that figure can increase up to 85%.

Not that we *ever* see faulty posture in the gym! After all, a guy squirming around on a machine trying to lift a weight he couldn't count to if he had a doctorate in math doesn't exactly exhibit what I'd call posture. He's just a dysfunctional mass of arms and legs writhing his way to the doctor's office. And even if he does manage somehow to get the weight up without his back exploding, with each

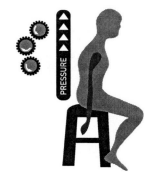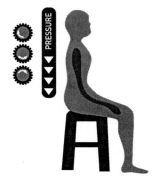

rep he increases his likelihood of incurring a serious orthopedic injury. He's playing favorites, allowing critical muscles to atrophy in comparison to others. No one has ever complimented him on his gracilis, so he only thinks in terms of quads and hams, or back and bi's, or chest and tri's. Whatever body part he's focused on, there are countless smaller muscles whose importance is being entirely overlooked—stabilizers and neutralizers.

CHAPTER 2:

STABILIZERS AND NEUTRALIZERS

One of the main problems with machine training is it usually works just the prime movers, the muscles primarily responsible for an action, with no consideration for the critical role played by stabilizers and neutralizers. What are stabilizers and neutralizers and why are they so important if you've never even heard of them?

Stabilizers—muscles which stabilize and/or support and protect a particular body segment while other muscles (prime movers) perform a movement. An example would be the action of the rotator cuff stabilizing the shoulder dynamically during the front crawl, thereby reducing the likelihood of impingement syndrome or "swimmer's shoulder." Of the body's 639 named muscles, it is interesting to note that nearly all play the role of stabilizer at one time or another.

Neutralizers—muscles which counteract unwanted and unnecessary movements of other muscles by producing an opposing action, thereby allowing for smooth, coordinated movements. A good example is the action of gluteus medius and minimus. Acting as medial rotators, they counteract the lateral rotation caused by an active gluteus maximus during the swing phase of running. If this lateral rotation is not neutralized, the gluteus maximus and the other lateral rotators may shorten and force will be reduced as they are no longer at an ideal length for hip extension. In addition, more energy must be used to medially rotate the laterally rotated leg in preparation for the swing phase of running. This all adds up to a less efficient stride and a slower run segment of a triathlon.

When the stabilizers and neutralizers are not trained in proportion to the development of the prime movers, a host of problems arise. Mike Clark, in part 7 of his *Essentials of Integrated Strength Training*, put it best when he said:

> *The nervous system is organized in such a way as to optimize the selection*
>
> *of muscle synergies and not the selection of the individual muscles. The*
>
> *nervous system thinks in terms of movement patterns and not isolated muscle*
>
> *function. Isolation and training individual muscles over prolonged periods of*
>
> *time creates artificial sensory feedback, faulty sensorimotor integration and*

53

abnormal forces throughout the kinetic chain. This ultimately acts to confuse the nervous system as muscles are being asked to perform a function that the nervous system does not understand.

Your muscles have a hard enough time with the demands you put on them attempting to swim, bike, and run all over the place. Now you want to make things worse by strengthening your favorite muscles while ignoring others. Aren't you familiar with the old adage about a chain and its weakest link? Do you need a newer analogy to understand what you're really accomplishing with all your misguided work in the gym?

Basically, you're building a souped-up engine and putting it in a Yugo. You may go real fast, but it handles like crap. It rattles over every bump in the road. And any time you go around a corner or slam on the brakes, a piece falls off. At first it's just the hood ornament (what is the Yugo emblem anyway?). Then it's a fender. And pretty soon the whole frame is in need of repair. How many triathletes do you know who are healthy throughout the entire season? I bet you some fuzzy dice for your Yugo that it's not many.

Yet every time you work out on the leg-extension machine at your gym, all you're doing is pimpin' up that Yugo. Yes, you're training your quadriceps—the prime mover in cycling and running. But you're training them in isolation. The antagonist muscles, the three muscles which compose the hamstring group, are being neglected. You are improving what is termed **intra-muscular coordination** or the capacity of your brain to recruit the motor units of your quadriceps.

One problem though. Outside of body building circles, the body rarely works in isolation. Even when you're lying comatose on the couch after a hard training session and performing twelve-ounce curls, you have stabilizers and neutralizers working alongside the prime movers flexing your elbow (not to mention the role your esophagus is playing). Machine-based training programs do a poor job of replicating the integrated fashion in which the body is made to function. The interaction of your stabilizers/neutralizers and agonists/antagonists—**your inter-muscular coordination**—gets completely ignored any time you exercise on those machines at the gym.

One of the key differences between movements and muscles is that the central nervous system knows nothing of muscles. In *Movement That Matters*, Paul Chek states that "during the constant adaptive changes that must take place while moving, the body is constantly activating an array of muscles in patterns of coordination, in which muscles lose their identity." In contrast, every time you work out on a machine, you're making a narcissist out of your quadricep or your hamstring. You're making those muscles big, dumb egomaniacs.

The quadricep that you've been training on the leg-extension machine allows both hip-joint flexion and knee-joint extension during running. Yet the hamstring, the poor middle child of your faulty exercise routine, has not learned to get along with the quad. You have been training it during the off season on the leg curl machine—in *isolation*. So when asked to function outside the familiar confines of the machine, the hamstring doesn't know how to act. Its normal function of restraining the extent of hip flexion and knee extension is overzealous, forcing its antagonist, the quad, to work more than is necessary. This costs you precious energy. In addition, in absence of sufficient hamstring activity, which would ideally generate tension at the same time as the quadriceps (and gluteals) to absorb the eccentric loading of the body's weight at footstrike, the tendons connecting these muscles to the pelvis are at risk of being overpowered.

Cancel your hotel reservations. You just tore a hamstring.

CHAPTER 3:
NEURAL DRIVE

The more stable a joint is (from proper stabilizer/neutralizer development), the more force a prime mover working on that joint can produce. Asleep on machines, the nervous system is awakened when exercising in the proper environment. Yet when stabilizers and neutralizers are not activated—a direct effect of training exclusively on machines—the prime movers are inhibited.

To further illuminate the point I'm trying to make, let's use a hypothetical example of a guy named Joe Pec Dec. Now, Joe spends so much time in the weight room that he probably gets his mail delivered there. In fact, the only time you don't see this guy in the gym is when the local tanning salon is running a two-for-one special. Mr. Pec Dec (and hypothetical or not, he's so much bigger than you and me, I suggest we refer to him as *Mister* Pec Dec) doesn't care one iota about stabilizers or neutralizers, and that's one of the reasons he trains on machines. Let's face it: His goal is to get freaking HUGE. A body-building competition doesn't give out awards for *function*. The requirements to grease the body down, step on stage, and flex individual body parts are elementary compared to the complex movements of swimming, cycling, and running in a triathlon. There is no need to:

- Condition stabilizers and neutralizers in relation to the prime movers

- maintain one's center of gravity over one's own base of support

- Integrate upper and lower extremity function

- Train **dynamic stability** as well as **static stability**

- Switch between **righting reactions** and tilting or **equilibrium reactions**

- Be proficient at both **closed** and **open-chain** movements (see Chapter Five of Section Two)

- Develop high levels of *inter* as opposed to *intra*-muscular coordination

It's analogous to learning to drive a car. When you were fifteen or sixteen, despite your transparent attempts to look like you were born with a driver's license, you had to really concentrate when behind the wheel. The distractions of light traffic, a person riding shotgun, or even a loud radio were detrimental to your mastery of driving (and hazardous to any mailboxes or trashcans that may have been positioned too close to the curb as well). You only had a certain amount of **neural drive** which you could allot to the task of driving.

57

But now you can sing to your favorite CD, put on make-up, talk on your cell, write down important messages, and eat a bowl of cereal—all while driving to work in rush-hour traffic. You've become, arguably, a better driver. You've reached the stage of autonomic development. You've got more neural drive to devote to the task of driving. Or, more specifically, being behind the wheel doesn't require as much of your neural drive as it once did. The process of driving a car now doesn't monopolize your concentration the way it did when you were a teenager. You've had years of driving in the real world, encouraging you to develop the skills necessary to function in that world. You've realized that if you want to go somewhere, you have to eventually take the car out on the road.

But bodybuilders aren't going anywhere. Their competitive environment is the stage—a uniformly level environment whose only real threat is the occasional drop of baby oil that doesn't get mopped up. Bodybuilders have the luxury of sitting down on a machine and concentrating solely on hammering out a set of eight to twelve with an obscene amount of weight. They can rely on the machine to:

- Act as their stabilizers and neutralizers

- Support their body

- Isolate upper or lower extremity function

- Nullify any need for dynamic or even static stability

- Minimize the demand of righting reactions with no need for tilting reactions

- Work primarily in an open-chain environment (sometimes a closed-chain one as well, but never both closed- and open-chain at the same time)

- Train isolated movements requiring little to no **inter**-muscular coordination.

With no need to think about anything other than flexing a specific muscle, bodybuilders can focus all their neural drive on making that muscle work. This allows them to lift more and more weight and, with the right combination of rest and *other* ingredients, get bigger.

Triathletes—and this probably goes without saying—are different. Most of us don't really care about bulging biceps or shredded pecs. We want to be fast, not big (the ripped quads are just a bonus). So if you want to be successful at this sport, it's time you got off that machine and went somewhere. And if you want to go farther than your driveway, working on correct stabilizer/neutralizer development is not only a good idea—it's essential.

Weak or untrained stabilizers can be overloaded quickly, sending inhibitory signals to the prime movers of a specific movement and resulting in *decreased* neural drive to those muscles. In other words, your nervous system will not allow the prime movers to fire at 100% of their capability *when they are not protected by the stabilization provided by the machine.* There is only one way to get around this problem and still follow the same machine-based gym protocol you've been doing for years. But I guarantee you that you'll be a heck of a lot slower coming out of T1 with your gym's leg press attached to your back.

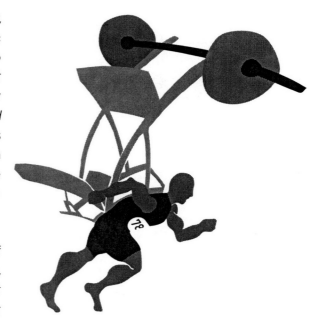

Your body is smart. It realizes when the structural integrity of the joint over which that muscle crosses is compromised, even if you don't. So you may be able to perform a squat on the Smith Machine with two hundred pounds. But your brain, just like when you were first learning to drive, won't allow you to utilize that power on the bike when your legs aren't guided through the motion like the thousands of reps you've performed in the past. There are just too many other things going on with which your machine-trained body is not familiar— like gravity, balance, and unguided motion. You simply will not be as strong on the bike as you thought. Strength training's detractors will cite this as evidence that lifting weights is of no benefit to the endurance athlete. And if you continue to lift incorrectly, the only thing you really end up strengthening is their argument.

Go prove it to yourself. After a couple of warm-up sets, do eight reps of a bench press at a weight which makes the last repetition a challenge. Have your training partner spot you to ensure we don't find your decaying carcass trapped underneath the bar a few days later. When finished, admire yourself in the mirror as you recover and stay loose for your next effort. Now, lie across a physio ball like like I'm doing in the FIGURE below and perform a set of dumbbell chest presses with the same amount of weight.

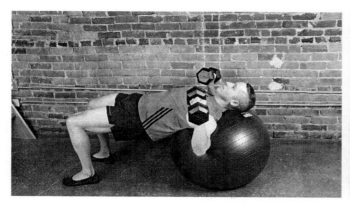
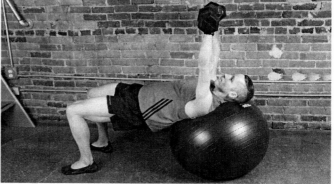

I doubt you could complete another set of eight. You may not have even been able to get the weight up off your chest. Don't feel bad. You just received a valuable lesson in neural drive which should feed your desire to train correctly. And if not, you can always get back on one of those machines and feed your ego!

Disproportionate development of prime movers in relation to stabilizers and neutralizers also changes the mechanics of joints. In the human body there are three classifications of joints or articulations: synovial, fibrous, and cartilaginous. These three can be further broken down into twelve subtypes, all of which share one common characteristic: They all are the points of contact between different bones. So if you change how a joint functions through an imbalanced exercise program (which is exactly the kind of program machine training lends itself to due to the inherent lack of stabilizer/neutralizer development), the result is the accelerated degradation of all the involved joint surfaces. Eventually you have bone contacting bone in places they were never meant to meet. The resulting liaison, despite all the anti-inflammatories in the world, can only end painfully.

In addition to the likely arthritic changes in a joint, overdevelopment of the prime movers in the absence of sufficient training for the stabilizers and neutralizers of the body creates a faulty **motor program**. Your body is like a computer. It stores the information on how to perform a given movement in what Richard Schmidt and Craig Wrisberg, in their book *Motor Learning and Performance*, term a generalized motor program. Yet each repetition of a movement performed on a machine essentially programs the computer with the wrong information. So stand up! Get off those machines. Turn your entire body on and program it with what it'll need to survive your next competition.

CHAPTER 4:

THE THREE DIMENSIONS OF LIFTING SUCCESS

Look at any decent book of kinesiology, and you'll learn that over 85% of our core musculature is oriented either horizontally or diagonally. We are built for rotation! Yet machines cannot accommodate us. Most machines are one-dimensional. They function in what is termed the **sagittal plane** (a vertical plane which divides the body into right and left halves—movement, therefore, occurs forward and backwards). The motion of the leg-extension machine, for example, takes place in the sagittal plane. Unfortunately, there are two other dimensions which get mostly ignored: the **frontal** (commonly referred to as **coronal**) **plane** (a vertical plane which divides the body into front and back—movement occurs side to side) and the **transverse plane** (a horizontal axis which divides the body into top and bottom—movement occurring here is rotational).

Ironically enough, these neglected planes of movement are the ones in which most people get injured. For example, most ankle injuries happen in the frontal plane while most knee injuries happen in the transverse plane. In a three-dimensional kinetic analysis of running, authors McClay and Manal concluded that "although relatively smaller than the sagittal plane component, a substantial amount of positive work was done in the frontal plane at both (the ankle and the knee), suggesting that this component should not be ignored."

Why would anyone conclude that training needs to include movements that don't directly contribute to forward propulsion? Well, if you train the body to be strong in only one plane of motion, it will not be strong enough to cope with the forces placed upon it in the other planes of motion. The inevitable result is injury. While the movements contributing to forward propulsion in triathlon do occur primarily in the sagittal plane, movements contributing to stabilization occur in the *transverse* and *frontal* planes. For example, the gluteus medius is dominant in the frontal plane. Thus, this plane of motion must be utilized when trying to target this muscle. But the weight training of the typical triathlete

SAGITTAL PLANE

CORONAL PLANE

TRAVERSE PLANE

BODY PLANES

63

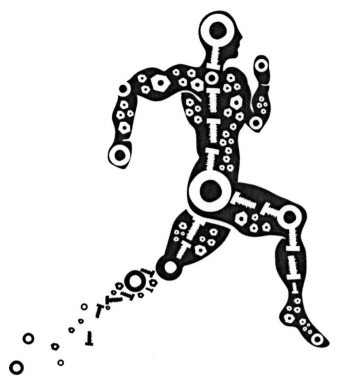

is sadly one-dimensional. And if the gluteus medius fails to activate sufficiently during the run, with each stride there is an excessive sideways motion of the pelvis toward the stance leg. This instability results in increased load on the knee or even the lumbar spine, not to mention a shorter stride. So as you swim, bike, and run, your Yugo chassis that you so tediously built in the gym with sagittal-plane-dominant lifting is falling apart. And you're going slower, to boot.

The movements which fail to prepare the body for all three planes of motion are fairly easy to recognize. Go into your local gym and look for the machines which have the manufacturer's name all over them. Typically, there will be a cushioned place to sit down on, and it'll probably be facing a mirror. If your gym is really busy, both of these characteristics will help explain the line of people waiting for their turn to work out on it. The pieces to which I'm referring and the dominant plane in which motion occurs are below:

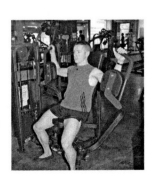

CHEST PRESS (SAGITTAL)

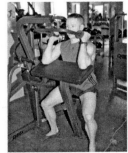

SEATED ROW (SAGITTAL)

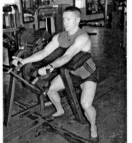

SHOULDER PRESS (SAGITTAL)

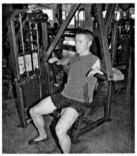

PEC DECK/FLY (SAGITTAL/FRONTAL)

TRICEP EXTENSION (SAGITTAL)

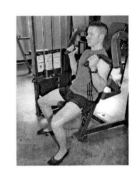

BICEP CURL (SAGITTAL)

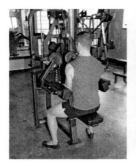

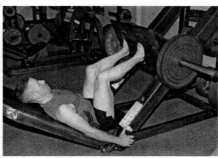

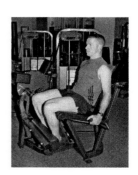

LATERAL RAISE (FRONTAL)   LEG PRESS (SAGITTAL)   LEG EXTENSION (SAGITTAL)

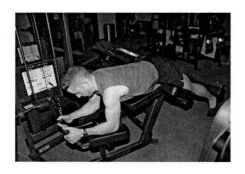

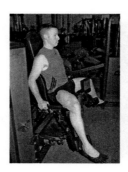

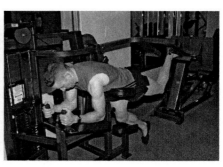

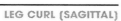

LEG CURL (SAGITTAL)   ABDUCTOR/ADDUCTOR (SAG/FRONT)   BUTT BLASTER (SAGITTAL)

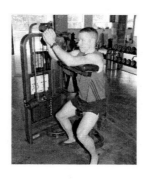

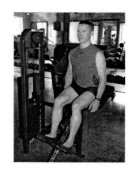

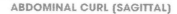

ABDOMINAL CURL (SAGITTAL)   BACK EXTENSION (SAGITTAL)

*NOTE that cable systems do not meet my definition of a machine, as they work in all three planes of motion and can often be utilized from a standing position—thus they get the Andrew stamp of approval.

Not only does your body find this one-dimensional, your mind does, too. In an article in *American Fitness*, Anita Goldman Horning quotes the athletic director of a local YMCA who says, "I haven't met anyone who was shown how to use the… machines once and couldn't use them on their own after that." This truth is *not* a badge of honor!

I remember going to Six Flags over Georgia when I was twelve. There was this one attraction where you "drove" these old fashioned cars around a track. I say "drove" because the track had a foot-high wall about two feet wide, which the cars straddled so that you could literally drive the car without touching the steering wheel. All you had to do was press on the gas pedal and the wall would guide the car around the track.

So I jumped behind the wheel with a buddy riding shotgun and a couple of my other friends in the car ahead. We had one speed: pedal to the metal—which for these cars translated to probably about eight miles per hour. But being a twelve-year-old boy, operating machinery, *and* without parental supervision, mind you, it was only a matter of time before I figured out how to get myself into trouble.

I made it half way around the track before my friends in the car ahead of me stopped. They looked back at me with mischievous grins, laughing about the road block they'd created. I laughed, too—not because they had stopped, but because I wasn't going to. Pulling myself up out of the seat, I hung onto the steering wheel and put all my weight into the gas pedal. Even at eight miles per hour, the collision was strong enough to jerk me off my feet, nearly sending me out of where the windshield should have been. Back on my feet, I looked back up at my friends' car in front of me and noted with satisfaction that it'd been slammed forward several feet. Then, glancing around to make sure none of the park authorities had noticed, I jumped back on the gas to ram them again.

This time I missed them. The car's wheels, which had been guided by the elevated center of the track, were now free. I pushed the gas down but forgot to think about steering and my car veered to the right. Before I could correct it, my vehicle was motoring along, at about a 7.5 minute/mile pace, toward the fence which separated the track from the rest of the park. *That* got the park personnel's attention. They came running from several directions, yelling at me to stop in voices with which my friends' raucous laughter and the rumbling engine couldn't compete. Something in their tones took the humor out of the situation and I immediately eased up off the gas. As the car coasted to a stop, I looked out the back at the new course my car had made. Two jagged scars cut across the landscape—it'd be my last ride of the day.

The simplicity of a machine-based exercise is its downfall. Sure, things work smoothly when you're guided by the pins, levers, and rails of a machine. But as soon as you're off track—which happens with your first step away from whatever piece you were working out on—your body no longer has any direction. You are literally moving in an environment for which you haven't adequately prepared yourself. And I'm writing as quickly as I can so I can get you back on course.

CHAPTER 5:

CLOSED CHAIN vs. OPEN CHAIN

One important concept to understand when looking at the deficits inherent to machine training is the difference between closed-chain and open-chain exercises.

Closed-chain exercises are movements in which the force applied is not sufficient to overcome the resistance so the BODY moves away from or toward the RESISTANCE. To put it simply, closed-chain exercises are ones in which the extremity is fixed and force is transmitted through the extremity. An example would be a squat or a pull up (even though the resistance is on the body during the squat, the force generated is applied to the ground and *not* the bar—and the bar is what ends up moving, *not* the ground).

Open-chain exercises are movements in which the force applied is sufficient to overcome the resistance so that the RESISTANCE moves away from or toward the BODY. In other words, the hands/feet are *not* fixed and can move freely. The leg extension or lat pull down are good examples of open-chain exercises.

Many human movements incorporate both closed- and open-chain aspects. Using you as our model, let's study the movements you make as you go through the three legs of a triathlon:

Swimming

With water 773 times more dense than air, you'd think it'd be easy to catch. But if you're an inefficient swimmer, instead of holding on to the water and pulling your body past your hand, you try to push the water away and behind you. You have made what should be a closed-chain activity an open-chain one. You end up swimming harder but not necessarily faster. Perhaps you should have done some more pull-ups to replicate the closed-chain aspect of the "catch." Only as your arm recovers should it be involved with an open-chain component. And seeing that up to 90% of your propulsion during freestyle swimming is created by the arms, if they aren't efficient in the water, you're in trouble.

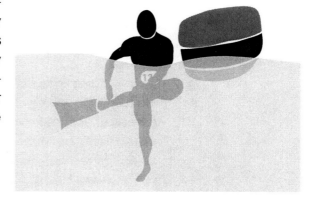

May I suggest you hide some fins at that first buoy.

69

Cycling

Open-chain movements predominate in cycling. The pedals are moving away from the body as you apply force to them (and toward the body, too, if you are also pulling up on the pedals instead of pedaling in squares). Admittedly, when you come to a hill significant enough to force you to stand, there is a brief instance when your body moves away from the pedals. At that moment, you are engaged in a closed-chain movement. But it soon reverts back to an open chain—unless you're too tired to pedal and stop moving your legs; and you fall over. But if you manage to keep the rubber side down, powering down the road in an aerodynamic tuck is an open-chain movement.

Running

As you apply force against the ground you move, so running is primarily a closed-chain exercise. Just as in swimming, the recovering limb (the leg in this instance) is involved in an open-chain movement, but your propulsion is delivered via your stance leg. Once again, you move, the ground doesn't—no matter how many Twinkies you ate over the off season!

But what about treadmill running? Ahh… now we come to a real "gray area" in the definition of closed vs. open chain. Strictly speaking, when running on a treadmill you are not moving but the belt is. So running on a treadmill is an open-chain exercise. And if you race on a treadmill, your run would probably benefit from open-chain exercises like a single-leg leg press. But I haven't been in a race yet where the organizers were ruthless enough to make me hop on a treadmill after a 112 mile bike and run a marathon. I'd probably drop out at T2 if they tried.

There's a race in San Francisco called The Escape from Alcatraz Triathlon. Second perhaps only to Kona in popularity, the event includes a critical section where you run on sand. You push against the sand and you move forward. But the sand moves underneath you, too—generally in the direction opposite of the one in which you have applied power via the stance leg. Proficiency, or at least familiarity, in open-chain or treadmill running is likely to be an advantage to the competitor here as the body makes the minute adjustments in sequencing and rate of power production necessary when ground reaction forces are different.

So how does knowledge of this concept impact your weight-training program for triathlon? Coupled with the fact that most machines are open-chain devices and numerous studies have consistently demonstrated that strength gains depend on the similarity between the training exercise and the actual physical performance being trained for, you can now eliminate those modalities with the least probability of transfer to triathlon. As one researcher states, "running involves the conversion of muscular forces into translocation through complex reciprocal movement patterns which incorporate nearly all of the major muscles and joints in the body" (Anderson, 1996, p.77). Now, does that sound even remotely similar to *any* machine you work on at the gym?

Machine training fails to replicate the mechanical demands of swimming or running. And the demands of cycling, where one is balanced precariously on a moving object with nothing to support the torso other than the strength of the rider's own musculoskeletal system, are impossible to mimic on something like a leg-curl machine. Yet triathletes by the hundred are rushing to *LIE DOWN*, grab a couple of handles to eliminate any possible core requirement, flex their knees so that their heels travel through the *sagittal* plane without a stabilizer muscle in sight, and kick themselves repeatedly in the butt.

The only thing even remotely sport specific about the whole thing is the ass-kicking they're destined to receive by any of their competitors who've read this book.

PATTERN OVERLOAD

Are you seeing a pattern here? If not, and you're still stubbornly working out on machines, your joints, ligaments, and tendons are beginning to see the pattern. And soon they'll feel it, too, in the form of what Paul Chek terms Pattern Overload. Literally trapped into the exact same range of motion rep after tedious rep, the muscles involved in any given machine based exercise— say a Smith Machine squat as opposed to a good, old-fashioned back squat—are unable to protect themselves by minutely changing the path of the bar as they would naturally do if performing an exercise allowing unguided movement in three planes of motion. The nervous system, in an effort to keep the fragile connective tissue from overload, as well as to conserve the body's limited supply of energy, wants to recruit different motor units at different times and at different rates during the lift. This ingenious protective mechanism not only prevents "overuse" injuries from occurring by avoiding the accumulation of micro-traumas brought on by the performance of identical movements. It also allows some motor units to rest while others are working.

Let's use the Ironman triathlon as a simple illustration of this idea. Taking anywhere from eight to seventeen hours to finish, the idea of this ultra-endurance event can have even the most focused, Type-A competitors among us intimidated and humbled by its demands. And even though we're triathletes—who, if our endless conversations about training schedules and aero gadgets are any indication, do not find many subjects tedious—at the end of the 2.4 mile swim, most of us are quite happy to get out of the water and do something other than use our arms over and over to propel our bodies through a sea of other athletes who can't seem to swim

71

a straight line. Then, after 112 miles on the bike, the thought of standing up to stretch our back, relieve the saddle pressure, and stop that incessant pedaling actually allows some competitors to look forward to running 26.2 miles. But it's realizing that each segment of the race will utilize a different movement pattern which makes the idea of tackling 140.6 grueling miles less daunting (admittedly, the obsessive-compulsive personality of the typical triathlete helps, too). Can you imagine what your arms would feel like if you had to swim the entire distance? Some of you more fish-like triathletes might say you'd welcome that. And even if that's true, you'd have some serious goggle marks which would take a solid week to fade.

But, getting back to the above example, squatting on the Smith Machine does not allow these slight variations to occur. Instead, the specific fibers of a muscle get worked the same way over and over again with each rep. And as these fibers begin to fatigue, the athlete's control over the movement deteriorates. The inevitable result is trauma to the muscle, connective tissue, and/or passive structures of the joint. And due to the avascular nature of tendons, ligaments, and collagen, the injury which results is slow in healing and often difficult to overcome without a cessation of training. While muscle tissue is nearly 100% healed after seven days, the connective tissue of your body may take six months to a year to recover fully. One study related this fact to triathlon, finding that triathletes have an injury rate of over 75%. In light of these figures, it's obvious that simply getting to the start line healthy is often the hardest part of triathlon!

To put it bluntly, I'll quote the authors of an article in a recent issue of the NSCA's *Strength and Conditioning Journal*:

> Short term studies using specific strength tests... have consistently indicated that free weights produce superior strength gains (than machines)... No studies could be located that indicated that machine training produces superior results in gains... These studies generally indicate the superiority of free weights in producing **a transfer-of-training effect.**

SPECIFICITY

The **Specific Adaptation to Imposed Demands (SAID)** principle of training dictates that the type of demand placed on the body controls the type of adaptation which will occur. And though only the activity being trained for provides 100% carryover to the event, the more closely an exercise resembles the activity, the higher the likelihood of usable *strength transfer.* Researchers Siff and Verkhoshansky refer to this transfer of training effect as "dynamic correspondence." They suggest a number of criteria that should be considered in selecting training modes in order to maximize this crossover from the gym to the competitive environment—most of which would be sorely limited by the confines of a machine.

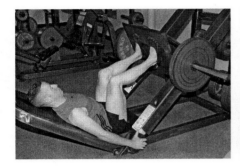 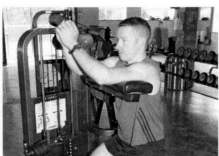 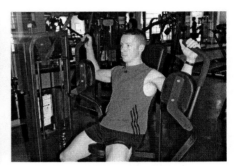

SWIM? BIKE? RUN?

Unless your definition of triathlon is leg press, ab crunch, and pec dec, you just can't come close to replicating the demands of multisport if you're exercising on machines. No, for a weight-training program to help you get faster at triathlon, the workouts prescribed require at least *some* neural output to design or perform. You need exercises which:

- Involve the actions of stabilizer and neutralizer musculature.

- Stimulate the nervous system.

- Are not guided or restricted but allow movement in all three planes of motion.

- Require use of your core musculature in a coordinated and integrated fashion.

73

CHAPTER 6:

MORE THAN "JUST ABS"

My clients have often heard me say that if people would activate their **transversus abdominus (TVA)** and learn to draw their navels in, we could solve the problem of world hunger. A bit of a stretch, I'll admit. And some would say politically incorrect, as well. But what I'm trying to stress is the importance of proper abdominal activation—in exercise, in sport, and in life.

It bears repeating: All movement emanates from or is coupled through the core. In fact, before you could even crawl you could move from one place to another. How'd you do that? Your mother probably asked that same question a hundred times by the time you were six months old. And, despite her exasperation, you twisted, squirmed, rolled and worked on developing the gross motor patterns of the trunk before mastering the fine motor skills of your extremities. This process, known as proximal-to-distal development, illustrates the essential role the core plays in the majority of movement patterns.

Yet despite their obvious importance, most people train their abs as an afterthought. They knock out a set of crunches at the end of their routine *if* they have the time. This backward thinking is perpetuated even by the so-called experts in the fitness community. The other day, I overheard a trainer laughing about his client who had chewed him out that morning for being five minutes late for their appointment. "The only thing she missed was abs," he said. "It's just abs!"

And that's the freaking problem today.

- If it was "just abs," then the incidence of back pain in people, as much as 80% by some estimates, would not be so prevalent.

- If it was "just abs," then more of us might actually be able to stand up straight, breathe properly, and save millions of dollars each year on unnecessary boob jobs and tummy tucks.

- If it was "just abs" then every elite athlete in the world, from Nicole DeBoom to Lance Armstrong, would spend "*only five minutes a day*" during their meticulous race preparation rocking back and forth on the newest version of the Ab Roller that they bought with just "*three easy payments of $19.95!*"

- If what that sadly typical trainer thought had any semblance of reality, and it truly was "just abs," then I really wouldn't have much to write about.

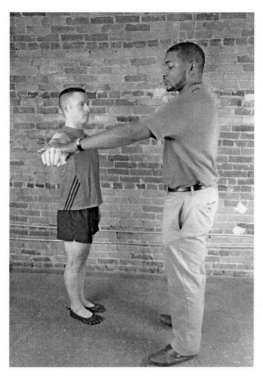

But I do.

Put your arm out to your side and hold it at shoulder level. Now get a training buddy to push your arm down as you resist, noting how much effort it took to move it. Then, try the same test again but activate your core by drawing your navel in toward your spine like you're trying to put on a tight pair of pants. Were you stronger on this second attempt? Your training partner may not have popped a blood vessel trying to get your arm down on either test, but I guarantee you he had to work harder the second time around.

Just abs...

If there is ANYTHING I want you to learn from this book, it is the importance of your core. **Improving your core function will go much farther *than any other training modality you employ* in your effort to become a better triathlete**. I highly recommend Paul Chek's *Scientific Core Conditioning and Scientific Back Training Series* as a resource to further your understanding of proper core development.

CHAPTER 7:

ABOMINABLE TRAINING ERRORS

Your abdominal-specific training should be placed last in your program so that the earlier exercises, *all* of which require proper activation and integration of the core now that you're not strapped into a machine, can be performed safely and efficiently. If your lower abdominals are fried, what's going to stabilize your lumbar spine when you're trying to knock out the last few reps of a 250-pound squat? So save the core-specific work for last, performing the more neurologically challenging or **axial loading** exercises first.

And while you're at it, skip all the crunches, too. In fact, I don't want you doing any crunches typical of most weight routines in this program. Not until you write me a thesis explaining how lying on my back with my knees bent and repeatedly picking my shoulder up six to eight inches off the ground for three sets of fifty reps is going to do anything to improve my triathlon performance.

Like the majority of my clients whom I have assessed in the past, most of you probably have adequate rectus abdominus strength. After years of crunch, sit-up, and leg-lift exercises done as the staple of abdominal programs since you were on training wheels, your upper abdominals are awake and functioning. Unfortunately, a muscle that was inadvertently conditioned at the same time is wired like an insomniac on No-Doze.

The psoas (pronounced SO-az—and you have two of them, originating on both sides of the last thoracic and all the lumbar vertebrae and inserting into the lesser trochanter of the left or right femur) is a muscle that becomes easily facilitated with improper or imbalanced abdominal training and the faulty posture which inevitably results. Together with the iliacus, they make up the hip flexors, with their primary action being to *flex* the hip.

Abdominal muscles do not cross the hip joint and cannot, therefore, create hip-flexion movements.

These hip-flexion movements condition the psoas and iliacus (as well as the rectus femoris and tensor fascia lata). When excessively developed from too many sit-up and leg-lift exercises, the hip flexors become exercise hogs, doing the work which should be accomplished by the lower abs and, thus, inhibiting them.

Inhibition of the lower abs is a common yet serious problem in both gym-goers and the sedentary population alike. As I said before, if you don't use it you will lose it. Despite what you might think, the body is inherently lazy. Even the triathlete's body, which we drag to the pool before dawn to punish with five thousand meters of hard swimming, will do as little work as necessary to function. So if your lower abdominals don't have to work, they ain't gonna work. And that's a big problem.

In contrast to the upper abdominals, the lower abdominals—those from the umbilicus down and innervated by the iliohypogastric and ilioinguinal nerves—are antagonistic to the lower back and, therefore, essential to the health and function of the lumbar spine. Florence Kendall, in her book, *Muscles Testing and Function*, says, "from the standpoint of good posture, the lower abdominals are more important than the uppers."

But if you've been training your abdominals improperly, the lower abs are probably fast asleep! And your back, not to mention your posture or your performance, is in jeopardy if you don't wake them up! Yet just *activating* your lower abdominal region requires coordinated and precise neurological control. They *must* be targeted *first*, before the complex movement patterns required to do them correctly become impaired by fatigue. The obliques should be trained next. And upper abdominal exercises, which involve simpler movement patterns, should be performed last or perhaps not at all until good motor control of the lower abdominals has been (re)established. Yes! You may actually need to *de-train* your upper abdominals to help balance out your muscular development and get your core functioning properly.

LOWERS before OBLIQUES before UPPERS

Like any other striated, skeletal muscle under voluntary control (as opposed to involuntary muscles such as *cardiac* muscle in the walls of the heart or *smooth* muscles in the walls of blood vessels or hollow organs), the abdominals need adequate recovery time between training sessions to repair. Think about it. Even our hypothetical Mr. Pec Dec, who couldn't *spell* abs if you asked him to, will tell you that you can't work your chest everyday, "you little girlie man!" So why do you work your abdominals daily? And Charles Poliquin, in his book *The Poliquin Principles*, states that the abs are actually fast-twitch muscles. Thus, they respond best to heavy-resistance, low-repetition sets. So I'll ask you another question—what are you really accomplishing with your three sets of one hundred?

High reps and inadequate recovery are a prescription for poor performance. Repeatedly breaking down your abdominals without allowing the necessary time for repair will eventually lead to adaptive shortening of this muscle group. As Chek notes in *Scientific Core Conditioning*, this common mistake can "disturb the normal respiratory excursion of the ribs, increase the workload on the accessory respiratory muscles, and encourage poor posture." Let that happen and your performance, inextricably linked to your posture, will suffer.

CHAPTER 8:

A POSTURAL TANGENT

Basic to an understanding of pain in relation to faulty posture is the concept that the cumulative effects of constant or repeated small stresses over a long period of time can give rise to the same kind of difficulties as a sudden severe stress.

—Florence Kendall

Posture is the position from which movement begins and ends. And as Paul Chek says, "If you begin in the wrong place you'll most likely end in the wrong place!" His pioneering course entitled *Scientific Back* Training paraphrases Kendall in defining *ideal* posture as:

> *that state of muscular and skeletal balance which protects the supporting structures against injury or progressive deformity, irrespective of the attitude in which these structures are working or resting. It is during a state of ideal posture that the muscles will function most efficiently.*

So what does this ideal posture look like? Well, you don't see it all that often, that's for sure, especially among the triathlon community. The combined effect of thousands of meters in the pool and hundreds of miles on the road, not to mention common weight-training errors, makes ideal posture among triathletes as rare as a Big-Foot sighting. It's a myth—the stuff of legends—with no sound basis in reality.

Until now.

Ideally, when viewed from the side, your ankle, knee, hip, shoulder, and ear should all line up (for a more detailed discussion of ideal postural alignment, see *Muscles: Testing and Function with Posture and Pain* by Kendall).

83

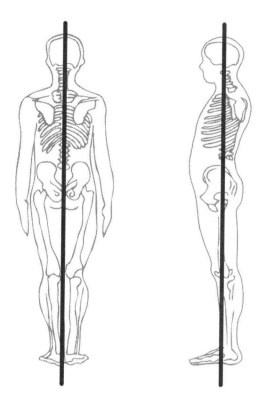

This alignment allows for the maintenance of proper length-tension relationships among your agonists/antagonist and neutralizers/stabilizers. But the body of the average triathlete does not exhibit these relationships. Typically, the body is out of balance—with short, tight pectorals and internal shoulder rotators coupled with long, weak scapular adductors. Fixed in what's termed a kyphotic position, with rounded shoulders and leading with their heads, triathletes *look* like they're on aero bars, even when they're not!

And as Kendall concludes, good alignment of the upper back is essential to good alignment of the head and neck. She continues:

Faulty alignment of the upper back adversely affects the head and neck position. If the upper back slumps into a rounded position in sitting or standing, there will be a compensatory change in the position of the head and neck.

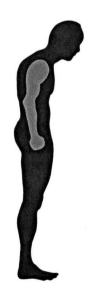

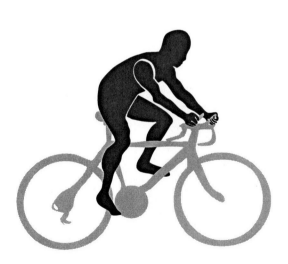

BIKE POSITION

BAD POSTURE

This compensation for excessive thoracic kyphosis occurs because the eyes will always seek the horizon. Literally programmed into our genetic code, this postural mechanism was essential for survival when we were cave men and women. If vision were compromised, your ability to avoid predators and other dangers suffered in kind. Admittedly, the threats in a triathlon are different. The lions and tigers have been replaced by potholes and Freds who can't swim or ride a straight line. But this same postural mechanism is still in play when racing or training. What do you have to do when you're time trialing on your aero bars and need to look forward? You extend your cervical spine! You flex the sub occipitals to bring your eyes up so they can see more than just your front wheel. But you don't leave your head in that position for 112 miles! That'd kill your poor neck muscles, and you'd have to run the marathon in a Peal Izumi neck brace.

Yet many triathletes are stuck in this kyphotic posture every waking hour—they've strengthened themselves in this position with hours of swimming, cycling, and running, so they now assume this posture training or not. Thus, those tiny muscles of the neck are burdened with the weight of the head, which as the lever arm increases, is magnified by that same weight for every inch it moves forward. Since the head weighs 7.5% of your body weight, this means the cervical musculature of a 150-pound triathlete with three inches of forward head posture is dealing with a head which effectively weighs *thirty-four pounds!!!* And no amount of carbo loading is going to make toting around that behemoth easy.

Can you say trigger points? I knew you could.

An additional consideration is that where the head goes the rest of the body follows. Compensations occur down the entire kinetic chain. So as the head travels forward, there will be a corresponding increase in the rounding of the upper back, with resulting changes to the lumbar spine, then the pelvis, to the knee, the ankle, and finally to the distal phalanges (five little piggies). Somebody's going to go "Wee! Wee! Wee!" all the way home.

Now your head's so far forward it's in a different time zone than the rest of your body. And your shoulders are rounded with the increased kyphosis of the thoracic spine making it look like you're wearing a Camelback. So what? You like the aero position. You have to race in it during triathlons, and practice makes perfect. This posture could only make you a better triathlete, right?

Let's break that argument down. And quickly, too, before your body gets broken down, as well. Muscles that are excessive in length are usually weak and allow for adaptive shortening of the opposing muscles. Muscles that are short are often strong and keep the weak, opposing muscles in a lengthened position. This perpetuates the orthopedic and/or functional problems associated with faulty posture. Applied to the triathlete above with the permanent aero position, we see the following:

Short and Tight: rectus abdominus, pec major, pec minor, anterior deltoids, upper trapezius, and sub occipitals.

Long and Weak: most muscles of the thoracic spine and anterior vertebral neck flexors.

Yup! What we got here is an old-fashioned muscle imbalance. And unless you take corrective action fast, you better hope your next triathlon is near Notre Dame because you'll soon be the spitting image of Quasimodo. But that's the least of your problems.

85

Try the following experiment:

Go stand in front of a mirror and face to the right or left so you have a side view of your body. Now take a big breath in. Then blow out all your air as hard as you can. Force every last bit of oxygen out of your lungs. Now check your image in the mirror and tell me what you see. Is your upper back rounded? Has your head come forward of your body? Do you look eerily similar to the aero-positioned triathlete we've been discussing?

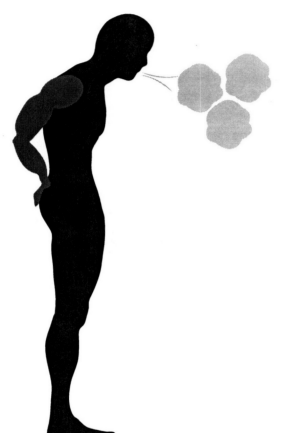

When you're stuck in this kyphotic posture that most triathletes assume, you are literally in a permanent position of exhalation. How can you expect to get the oxygen *in* when you're fixed in a posture better suited for blowing that oxygen *out*? With these altered respiratory patterns, your aerobic capacity is diminished by as much as a third. And, excuse me, but the last time I checked, triathlon was primarily an aerobic sport. Breathing correctly is essential to success. You cannot afford this aerobic deficit—it's costing you places in your age group. It may even be costing you your rightful place on the podium.

Kendall says that "the position of the pelvis is the key to good or faulty postural alignment." If this is true, then in order to improve this exaggerated curvature of the thoracic spine, you must also address the muscles which influence the position of the pelvis. That's right. Excessive kyphosis of the upper back is not your only problem.

CHAPTER 9:
PELVIC TILT

Cycling works the quads—ninety times per minute, per leg. That equates to 27,000 reps per leg during the course of a five-hour Ironman bike leg. So is it any surprise that your quads are in need of stretching? Combine this fact with an imbalanced core-training program which leaves the iliopsoas short and tight and the lower abs long, weak, and doing their best impression of Rip Van Winkle, and you've set the table for a pelvis with too much anterior tilt.

Never heard of **anterior pelvic tilt**? Not too worried about it? Well, because the thoracic spine is affected by the position of the low back, increased anterior pelvic tilt can lead to excessive lumbar lordosis which, in turn, contributes to even more rounding of the upper back. Still not concerned? Maybe you're a fan of dowager's humps? Well, what if I explained to you how increased pelvic tilt can slow your swimming and wreck your running?

PELVIC TILT AND SWIMMING

89

There are two simple ways to swim faster:

increase your stroke rate (SR)
or
increase your stroke length (SL)

In other words, SR x SL = swimming velocity. But Terry Laughlin, founder of Total Immersion, holds that increasing SR is self-limiting because energy cost goes up by a cubic relationship. Taking your SR from two times per second up to four times per second results in you burning through your limited energy supplies eight times faster (2 x 2 x 2 = 8). Laughlin goes on to state that "faster swimmers take fewer strokes than slower swimmers—at every level from Olympic finals to lap time at the local Y."

But if your pelvis is tilted anteriorly (a condition exacerbated by the tight lats which result from lots of pool time) and your upper back assumes a position of kyphosis, the short, tight muscles of the pectorals and deltoids will inhibit your reach, thus decreasing stroke length. The only way to make up for this deficit is to increase your turnover, which costs you energy you cannot spare.

In addition, the forward head carriage associated with a kyphotic posture puts your melon deeper in the water and greatly increases drag. Ask the best swim coaches in the world and they'll tell you that reducing drag will produce greater dividends

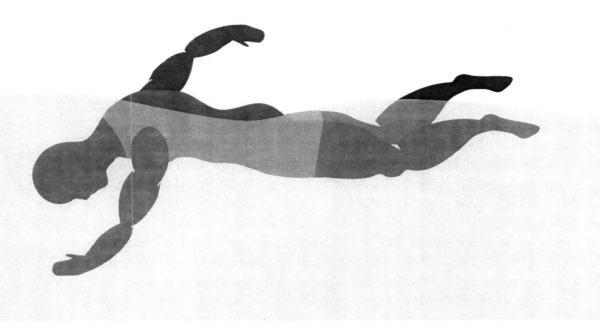

in the water than anything else you can do. You want to swim through the smallest cylinder possible. But that's hard to do when your cranium is virtually scraping the lane line at the bottom of the pool while your upper back breaks the surface of the water like the dorsal fin of a shark.

That's some serious drag you're creating. And it's all because of your faulty posture. In addition, if you cannot extend the thoracic spine because you're stuck in a position of kyphosis, every stroke you take will put excessive strain on the muscles and connective tissue of the shoulders. As the prime movers involved in swimming become fatigued and their movements become less efficient, the four tiny muscles of the rotator cuff become overworked in an attempt to dynamically stabilize the glenohumeral joint. Ten thousand meters a week later, you've developed a nice case of swimmer's shoulder.

When defined as "significant shoulder pain that interferes with training or progress in training," 35% of elite and senior level swimmers report episodes of swimmer's shoulder. What they are experiencing may not technically be swimmer's shoulder but a similar condition called thoracic outlet syndrome. The thoracic outlet is the space between clavicle and rib cage through which nerves and vascular structures pass from the neck and thorax to the arm. The symptoms of thoracic outlet syndrome are similar to swimmer's shoulder and numerous other clinical diagnoses, but they all have one thing in common. As Kendall states, "treatment should emphasize increasing the space of the thoracic outlet by improving the *posture* (and) correcting the *muscle imbalance*... that adversely affect the posture of the head, neck, and upper back." (Italics mine.)

PELVIC TILT, PRONATION AND RUNNING

As in swimming, above, there are two ways to increase running speed:

increase stride rate (SR)
or
increase stride length (SL)

Therefore, running velocity (RV) can be illustrated as SR x SL = RV. Lengthening your stride by just one inch "shortens" the marathon at the end of the Ironman by one kilometer, as the number of strides to cover the distance decreases. This translates into a finishing time five minutes faster for the runner finishing the marathon in 3.5 hours. The gains for slower marathoners would be even greater. Yet stride length is shortened in athletes with too much anterior pelvic tilt as hip flexion becomes limited. This position of the pelvis also increases ground-contact time, an undesirable aspect for improvements in speed. And dangerous, too—after all, you don't get injured in the air!

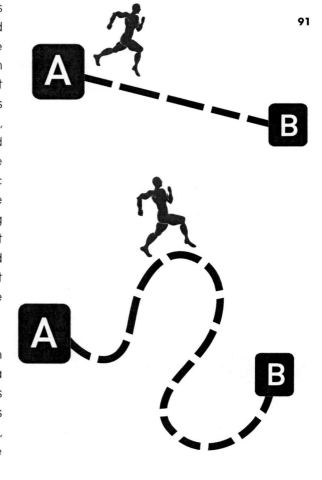

NOTE: With the preceding paragraph's focus on the performance detriments of a shortened stride length, one might conclude that I place less importance on the effect of stride rate on running speed. However, it is my experience that most runners overstride. That is, the foot lands heel-first in front of the athlete's center of mass, creating both a braking effect and increased sheer force up the kinetic chain. This is undesirable from both a performance and an orthopedic standpoint. In essence, the athlete is using more muscle mass (and, thus, more energy), creating more vertical oscillation (and, thus, more impact upon landing), going up rather than forward, and ignoring a simple rule of physics—the shortest distance between two points is a straight line (see FIGURE).

While it can destroy your finishing time, running with excessive lumbar **lordosis** can be even more of a problem for your orthopedic health. Anterior pelvic tilt is associated with **femoral anteversion** which predisposes the athlete to a host of pronation injuries. Shin splints, iliotibial band syndrome, and patellofemoral syndrome are all prime examples of preventable injuries which ruin the seasons of countless promising triathletes.

During the first half of the support phase of running, the increased load on the subtalar joint causes it to pronate faster and with greater magnitude than that which normally occurs with walking. This leads to increased tibial internal rotation which is transmitted to the knee, forcing the knee to collapse medially. Couple that with the increased femoral anteversion caused by excessive anterior pelvic tilt and you have a hip, or a knee, or an ankle in a position in which it was never meant to be.

There is an indisputable fact that force is transmitted best through a straight line. So as you run all catawampus with a knee over here and a hip way over there, not only are you losing potential speed—with every stride you're hastening the demise of your athletic career. You are tearing your body up. Think about what you learned in high-school physics class: For every action there is an equal and opposite reaction. Thus, pushing on the ground results in the ground pushing back at you. Yet your body is not aligned properly. So just like when you fail to hammer a nail straight down and the nail bends, each misaligned step you take not only robs you of propulsive force. It also brings you that much closer to the breaking point. And if you just came home with a sweet new pair of motion-control shoes from your local running store to eliminate this problem, sneakers aren't the only thing they sold you. You just bought into what the shoe companies have been selling to the running community for years: the idea that **pronation** is an evil word.

Yet pronation (a combination of dorsiflexion, calcaneal eversion, and internal rotation—refer to left Figure) is how the body absorbs shock. And its opposite motion, **supination** (plantar flexion, calcaneal inversion, and external rotation—again, see left Figure), is how the foot acts as a rigid lever for forward propulsion.

Too little pronation not only forces the knee to endure rotational stresses it was not designed to handle (after all, the decreased motion of the foot must be made up somewhere); it also transfers too much of the landing impact to the rear of the foot. Try the following

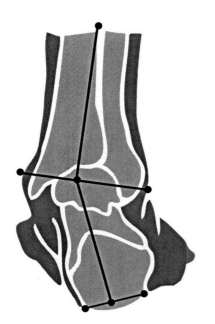

REAR VIEW OF LEFT FOOT SUPINATION

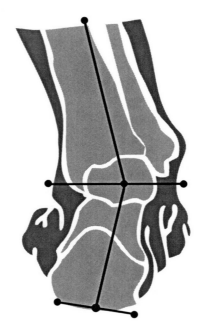

REAR VIEW OF LEFT FOOT PRONATION

experiment I learned at one of Joe Friel's Endurance Coaching seminars in Boulder, Colorado:

Stand up and begin hopping on the balls of your feet with your legs straight. Feel the springiness in your feet and calves. It's effortless. Given a good Tour de France video, some power bars, and perhaps a dare you accepted while in a drunken stupor and you could jump like this all day.

Continue jumping. But, now, switch to landing on your heels. Do you feel the difference? The impact forces can literally be felt all the way up to your skull. Can you imagine landing like this for 26.2 miles? But if you've been told you over-pronate and should wear special, beefed-up shoes or even orthotics to control excess motion in your feet, you're not allowing the natural shock absorbers of your body to work.

Why are you treating the *symptom*? Why not treat the *source* of the problem?

Let's examine how the position of the pelvis influences the movements of the lower leg. Stand up and tilt your pelvis forward or anteriorly and you'll feel your weight shift forward and to the insides of your feet (pronation). Now tilt your pelvis backward or posteriorly and you'll feel your weight shift backwards and to the outsides of your feet (supination).

93

Martin and Coe, the authors of Training Distance Runners, say that "although it is the foot that strikes the ground, the actual pivot point for the lever system that provides movement is really the lumbar spine and pelvis."

The source of the problem of excessive pronation may very well be your pelvis.

You can control excessive pronation by controlling excessive anterior pelvic tilt. To do that, you need an exercise program which will strengthen the muscles of the force couple which pull the pelvis up in the front and down in the back. In addition, you may need to stretch the muscles of the force couple which pull the pelvis up in the back and down in the front. Specifically:

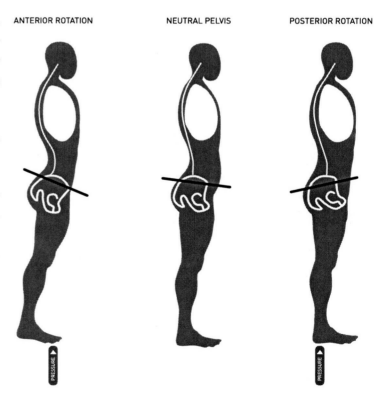

ANTERIOR ROTATION   NEUTRAL PELVIS   POSTERIOR ROTATION

STRENGTHEN: lower abdominals, gluteals, and hamstrings.

STRETCH: latissimus dorsi, lumbar erectors, iliopsoas (hip flexors), and quadriceps.

Of course, there are cases when a properly made pair of orthotics is necessary for an athlete, such as when the metatarsal heads have dropped and the athlete does not accept load into the forefoot efficiently. But many of these biomechanical abnormalities have etiologies which are rooted in core dysfunction or length/ tension imbalances. All too often, these basic faults at the very least hasten the onset of a condition which will ultimately require medical intervention.

CYCLING AND PELVIC POSITIONING

And lest you erroneously begin to think cycling is one sport where your orthopedic health is unaffected by posture, let's examine the pedal stroke and the demands it places on the body.

As a cyclist pedals, the majority of force production is provided by the quadriceps, which extend the knee approximately 74° from 111° flexion to 37°. During extension, the knee also adducts due to the normal valgus angulation of the distal femoral condyles in relation to the foot/pedal interface during the downstroke. This causes medial translation of the knee as it extends. In addition, pronation of the foot coupled with internal tibial rotation increases stress on the medial knee. Sounds like a recipe for overuse, doesn't it? Yet that's what happens during the normal pedal stroke! These are the biomechanics of a healthy cyclist!

The flexibility and strength imbalances which can both result from or be the cause of faulty pelvic alignment can literally tear up the knees of the posturally challenged cyclist. Tight quads, hams, iliotibial bands, or any other muscle with a restricted range of motion can increase the forces on the tibiofemoral joint. And as you pedal at ninety revolutions per minute, the repetitive forces across the knee are magnified when weakness in any of the muscles that comprise the leg leads to fatigue-induced alterations in pedaling technique. I don't know about you, but I'm pretty baked toward the end of a five-hour ride. I'm starting to feel those 27,000 pedal strokes! Now, do you really want to add postural faults to the mix and increase your chances of leaving random parts of your knees out on the road somewhere?

95

CHAPTER 10:

THE INNER UNIT AND BACK PAIN

Another problem with too much anterior pelvic tilt is that it can lock up the lumbar facet joints, not allowing proper rotation of the lumbar spine. Not only does this impair swimming and running performance (both sports which require a complementary rotational component), it can also irritate the facet joints and the anterior longitudinal ligament of the lumbar spine. The facet joints are fed by the same nerve which reflexively innervates an important muscle in spinal stabilization called the **multifidus**. Since pain inhibits function, and the multifidus is on the same neurological loop as the transversus abdominus, pelvic floor musculature, and the diaphragm, all these key players in what Australian researchers Richardson, Jull, Hodges, and Hides term the **Inner Unit**, will be inhibited and will not work properly.

When this happens, you have a "naked spine" which cannot withstand the impact forces that occur during training or racing. Rick Jemmett, author of *Spinal Stabilization*, notes research which concludes that even the strongest region of the spine can tolerate only nine kilograms (approximately twenty pounds) of stress before failing under the load and becoming injured. Now consider that impact forces incurred during running can increase to as much as six times body weight. For a 150-pound runner moving at a six-minute-per-mile pace, with a cadence of ninety foot strikes per minute, this amounts to 486,000 pounds of cumulative impact force *per foot per mile!* My back hurts just thinking about it.

And I don't want to go through back pain again. Been there. Done that. In 2002, I was involved in a pile up of twelve guys or so during the Tuesday-night training criterium in Atlanta. A guy I coached, who could have obviously benefited from some bike-handling lessons, overreacted to a small crash ahead of us, locked up his rear wheel, and fell off his bike. Luckily, I was there to cushion his fall. 175 pounds moving at twenty miles per hour hit me from the side, and I was pinned by bikes and rider before I could say uncle.

Not too happy, I got up, delivered some choice expletives, and did the first thing that any true cyclist would do—I checked to see if my bike was okay. The rear derailleur hanger was torn off and the front wheel taco'd. And then, as I looked down at the road rash on my arms which was just beginning to ooze, I realized the worst part: My wife was going to kill me!

The reason I got into triathlon in the first place was because my wife asked me to

97

give up cycling after a crash in a domestic criterium resulted in my third concussion. Apparently she didn't like being woken up in the middle of the night to be told by a nurse that her husband was in an emergency room five hundred miles away. And the slurring of my words and short-term-memory loss were probably not terribly attractive either. That I had lost my equilibrium and had to learn how to ride a bike all over again scared her a bit, too, I'm sure.

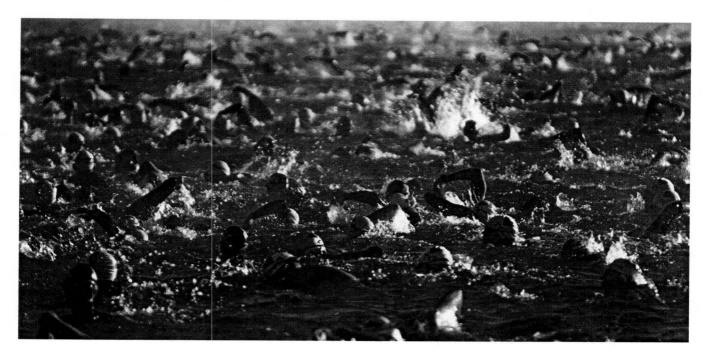

But I convinced her that triathlon was safer. After all, she comes from a swimming background, with convenient little lane lines and eight polite people sharing a pleasant day at the pool. There was no way she could ever imagine two thousand Kona-crazed triathletes all competing for the straightest line to the first buoy marker. So, I retired from competitive cycling and promised her I'd ride alone if she just wouldn't take my bike away.

And now she was going to know the truth.

That fear was probably why I didn't really notice the pain in my lower back as I carried my tangled bike back to the car. I was too preoccupied with thoughts of marital disaster to realize that my back, like my wheel, was out of true. I had a serious injury, later diagnosed as a bulging disc and sprained SI joint, with immediate and long-term consequences.

The multifidus, a key member of the Inner Unit which usually protects a spinal joint, doesn't activate properly when injured and quickly atrophies—as much as 25%

in twenty-four hours—with the dysfunction continuing even after the symptoms of pain have disappeared. This occurs because, unlike many other muscles with polysegmental innervation (i.e., more than one nerve root to deliver commands), the multifidus has unisegmental innervation. This means it has, in effect, one brain. As a result, this tiny muscle has no back-up nerve to feed it in case of injury. If the multifidus shuts down, the part of the spine which it stabilizes is at the mercy of every impact force transmitted through the body.

Speaking of impact forces, a week after the crash I raced an Olympic distance tri on Monday, a sprint on Saturday, and a half-Ironman on Sunday. I ended up winning them all. But with my multifidi on an extended lunch break, the L5/S1 segment of my spine had nothing to stabilize it, nor anything with which to dissipate the loads I encountered during the course of those three races. My pain got progressively worse until, literally five minutes after crossing the finish line of the half-IM, I couldn't walk. My season was over.

To explain what happened, here's some basic anatomy. The human spine consists of twenty-five individual bones called vertebrae (including the five fused portions of the sacrum and the coccyx) which are connected by spinal discs, ligaments, and, fortunately, muscles. Contrary to popular belief, the spine by itself was not meant to be a weight-bearing structure. If it were, then most buildings would be shaped like an S and elevators would be a lot more fun to ride. No, your spine is actually quite delicate. And its long-term health is predicated on the proper conditioning and sequencing of specific musculature to stabilize it, which traditional core-training programs fail to do.

Let's use a politically incorrect analogy to illustrate this concept. The L5/S1 disc is Martha Stewart. Her home is the spinal column made up of twenty-five bricks (the vertebrae) held together with mortar (muscles of the Inner Unit). And the ankle bracelet she wears while under house arrest is the nervous system which communicates the position of all the above anatomy. So one day a tornado hits. It's a severe storm, enough to weaken the mortar serving the L5/S1 "bricks." But the problem is ignored, so the mortar becomes weaker with each successive thunder shower causing more damage to it. Then one day, after three storms in a week (on a Monday, Saturday, and Sunday), the mortar cracks and allows the L5 and S1 bricks to move. Martha Stewart quickly escapes and the ankle bracelet fails to relay the information to the authorities until it's too late. Martha's gone. The disc has bulged, and now I have to endure rampant insider trading and cheesy floral arrangements (my somewhat stretched analogy for pain).

Paul Chek defines "dynamic stability" as "the ability to maintain an optimal instantaneous axis of rotation in any joint or combination of joints in any space/time

99

combination." He goes on to say that "dynamic stability requires that each joint complex in the body be stabilized by its respective stabilizer muscles in such a way that it functions within the parameters necessary to maintain optimal joint health." You can safely say that my dynamic stability was lacking after I crashed. I was in pain. And since pain inhibits function, my multifidi weren't working properly. This meant the other components which make up my Inner Unit and are on the same neurological loop as the multifidi were probably not functioning properly either. My spine was as naked as an exhibitionist at a nude beach.

The other crucial member of the Inner Unit is the transversus abdominus (TVA). The TVA is the deepest of the four abdominal muscles and its importance is highlighted by the fact that it is the only abdominal muscle which attaches directly to the spinal joints. I tell my clients that it is the weight belt you were born with. Its fibers are positioned in the transverse plane, so activation of this muscle brings the navel in toward the spine, acting like a girdle (i.e., weight belt) to flatten the abdominal wall and compress the abdominal viscera. This creates what is referred to as *hoop tension*. As the umbilicus is drawn in against the non-compressible abdominal viscera, a stabilizing effect on the lumbar spine is created.

But many triathletes have convinced themselves they need to buy a weight belt instead of using the one they've had all their lives. After all, the more seasoned gym veterans—the ones slamming the weights around and grunting like pregnant heifers—they wear them. They didn't spend any time and energy to build their weight belts. They just charged one to their Am Ex, took it to the gym, cinched it down so tight their eyes bulged in their sockets, and started lifting!

The problem with strength training while wearing a weight belt is that it leads to faulty activation of the core. The way in which the weight belt creates hoop tension beyond that created by the exerciser tightening the belt is the exact *opposite* of how the body was designed to stabilize the spine. The fibers of the rectus abdominus and external oblique fire *away* from the spine—opposing the activation of the TVA. They push into the belt as the load increases. And while this does increase gross stability of the spine, it leaves the spine unprotected at the segmental level.

Then what happens when you're not wearing the belt? When you're... say... racing in a triathlon? Now you've programmed your body to fire the rectus abdominus and external oblique under load. You've allowed your deep abdominal wall, your TVA and internal oblique, as well as the other members of the Inner Unit to become detrained. You have, through facilitating your rectus abdominus and ignoring the development of the weight belt you were born with, allowed faulty recruitment patterns to ingrain themselves in your neuromuscular system. Essentially, you have programmed your computer with the wrong information. If proper core activation is an essential component to the performance and orthopedic health of an athlete, as I maintain it is, then you have decreased your chances of making it through the triathlon season injury-free.

BOTTOM LINE: The only time you should be wearing a belt in the gym is if you need one to hold your pants up.

It takes five hundred days for a disc to heal fully. So with time and an exercise program that targeted the multifidi and TVA, I was able to return to the competitive arena. And while the time in between was both frustrating and painful, it allowed me to delve further into the world of corrective exercise. Unable to pursue my athletic endeavors, I opted for academic enrichment. In fact, many of my physical setbacks could, in hindsight, be seen as career opportunities. But, like many of you who are reading this while sidelined because of injury, I would much rather have been racing.

Yet the odds seem stacked against us. Some researchers hold that as many as 80% of adults will experience back pain at some point in their lives. And, according to a study by C.M. Bono, degenerative conditions which often cause back pain are more prevalent in athletes than the sedentary population. After all, most athletes aren't aware that they even *have* an Inner Unit. And the couch potatoes among us couldn't care less.

Until it's too late.

THE STRENGTH OF THE WORKOUTS

Strength is one of the most important biomotor abilities, and its role in an athlete's training is often paramount. Understanding the methodology of its development is primary because it affects both speed and endurance.

—Tudor Bompa

CHAPTER 1:

The Anatomical Adaptation Phase (AA)

You're going to be sore. That's inevitable. Anytime you perform a new movement or have an extended break away from training, your body is going to let you know that it's not familiar with the demands you're placing on it. Typically appearing 24-72 hours after the training stimulus, this pain and stiffness, referred to as **delayed-onset muscle soreness**, or **DOMS**, usually diminishes within five to seven days.

But muscular recovery is not a grave concern. Muscle has a good blood supply. Like oil is to your car, blood is to the body. The sore muscles will recover. It's the connective tissue, the tendons and ligaments, which dictate the parameters during this phase of weight training.

The reps are high so that the intensity will be low, giving the connective tissues time to heal from the trauma incurred during lifting (which is minimal due to the comparatively light loads employed). Don't confuse high *density* training with high-intensity training. Repetitions and load are inversely proportional. As one goes up, the other comes down. Think about it. How many times can you get up from a chair, sit back down, and then get up again? A lot! It's low intensity. You may get some strange looks from anybody in the room, but you're an athlete—you could do this all day. Now how many times could you sit in that same chair and get up again if you had to do it holding a brand-new 50" plasma TV? It'd be a lot fewer, and not just 'cause the tour is on OLN. It's heavier. The load (i.e., the intensity) is a lot higher, so you can't do as many reps. Better hope that chair's a comfortable one.

103

In comparison to muscle, connective tissue heals much more slowly. It can take as much as seven times longer to heal due to a comparatively meager blood supply in contrast to muscle. Also, tendons and ligaments contain fibers which are less elastic than muscle tissue and therefore are more subject to injury without proper preparation.

And that's what this cycle of lifting is all about—preparation of the muscles, of the fragile connective tissue, and of the athlete's neuromuscular system. In fact, during the first four to six weeks of a new training plan, gains in strength are mostly neural. The muscles are getting smarter. Since the loads used in this phase are relatively low, the athlete can focus on form and technique. This is of the utmost importance due to the **Law of Facilitation** which states:

When an impulse has passed once through a certain set of neurons to the exclusion of others, it will tend to take the same course on a future occasion, and each time it traverses the path the resistance in the path will be smaller.

In laymen's terms this means that every time you perform a repetition of an exercise incorrectly, it becomes easier and easier to do that movement incorrectly and more difficult to perform the right way. In my training at the CHEK Institute, I have learned that it takes as little as three hundred repetitions to learn a specific movement. But if you've been performing an action with a faulty motor program because you never learned how to do a specific movement correctly, it can take as many as five thousand repetitions to program your brain with the right information. Remember:

QUALITY IN = QUALITY OUT!

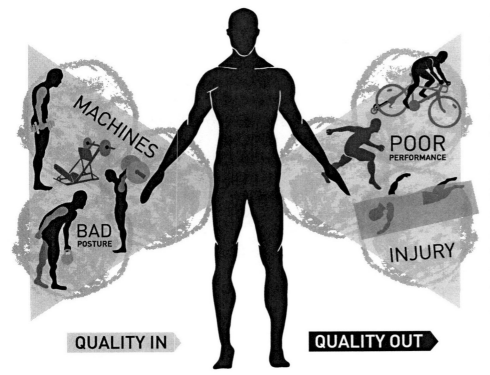

The high repetitions during this training phase serve another purpose as well. Consider the six-to-twelve repetition pattern commonly employed in many people's strength-training programs. This rep scheme is perfect for muscle hypertrophy, a goal of many gym enthusiasts. At an average of two seconds for the concentric phase and two seconds for the eccentric phase, the average repetition lasts only about four seconds. Multiply that by six to twelve, and you have an average set time of twenty-four to forty-eight seconds. And that's being overly optimistic, as it is my experience that most gym-goers lift on a 1-0-1 tempo. That equates to twelve to twenty-four seconds of **time under tension**. Thus, the energy used to achieve maximal effort in this time frame comes primarily from anaerobic sources.

Anaerobic means "without oxygen." Without oxygen, the body does not optimally provide the muscles engaged in a given movement with some of the adaptations crucial to success in a triathlon, specifically increased capillary density. This lack of vascular development in a muscle whose cells have grown in size and volume results in an environment which is ischemic. As the muscle tissue becomes anemic due to the diminished supply of oxygen and other nutrients, crucial metabolic processes, including the elimination of waste products created during exercise, slow down. Ultimately, this results in premature fatigue. And as mentioned above, the risk of damage to connective tissues is even greater due to the compromised supply of blood to these tissues. Neither of these outcomes is beneficial in a triathlete's quest for the finish line.

No wonder there's so much debate about whether strength training benefits the endurance athlete. If the subjects in a particular study are getting heavier; if they are increasing muscle mass without a corresponding increase in adequate blood flow to the working tissues; and if all the "studies" are utilizing movements which have no transfer of training effect to sport in general, then the only conclusion which can be drawn from the inevitable and obvious results is that weight training sucks!

"Time under tension" is the key concept of the Anatomical Adaptation phase. The twenty-to-thirty reps utilized for the majority of exercises performed during this first of five training periods increases the time under tension to 80-120 seconds (20-30 repetitions x 4 seconds = 80-120 seconds). Contrasted with the typical twelve-to-twenty-four seconds it takes to complete the repetitions in a typical program, this stimulates greater capillary density in and around the working muscle as production of ATP (adenosine triphosphate) becomes more dependent on oxygen and less on other fuel systems (i.e., the ATP/CP system or the fast glycolytic system). Now the environment in the body is optimized for recovery and regeneration. Better recovery leads to an athlete who can more easily withstand the demands of the next training cycle, the next workout day, or even the next swim stroke. Thus, the Anatomical Adaptation phase lays the foundation for the triathlete's strength-training program; appropriately, it is also the phase to which the intelligent triathlete returns in a properly periodized program to increase the likelihood of a successful season.

Anatomical Adaptation Phase Details

- *Circuit training*—Do one set of exercise #1 and then do one set of exercise #2, etc., progressing to the next exercise as quickly as possible. KEEP MOVING!

- 2-3 circuits (third set added only after workout can be accomplished without post-exercise soreness)

- If possible, choose a different exercise each set to expose the body to different movements

- 90 seconds between circuits

- 20-30 reps

- 2-3 days a week on non-consecutive days

- Use every fourth week as a recovery week by cutting out one circuit of weight training

- Always perform exercises with higher **neurological demand** and/or **axial loading** earlier in the workout

- 45-60 minutes approximate workout time

> **1. Leg Exercise from Squat, Lunge, or Bend pattern**
>
> **2. Pull-Pattern Exercise**
>
> **3. *Non-axial-loading* leg exercise**
>
> **4. Push-Pattern Exercise**
>
> **5. Pull-Pattern Exercise**—*use a different exercise than #2 above.*

THESE FIVE EXERCISES SHOULD BE PERFORMED IN A CIRCUIT FASHION. FOLLOWING COMPLETION OF THE FINAL CIRCUIT, RESERVE APPROXIMATELY FIFTEEN MINUTES FOR THE FOLLOWING:

Back-Extension (found in the BEND PATTERN section)—preferably on an unstable surface like a Swiss Ball (Ex. Prone Cobra, Alternating Superman, Reverse Back-Extension, etc.)

Abdominal—lowers before obliques before uppers (if you do uppers at all—commonly the most developed in people). Again, employ unstable surfaces and a variety of exercises.

Exercises (circuit 1)	Sets	Rest	Reps	Intensity	Tempo/ Duration
Front Squat Maintain lordosis, TVA activation and knees over toes	1	n/a	20-30	2 RR	Moderate
Pull-Ups (with assistance) Keep hips underneath shoulders (i.e., don't allow pelvis to sway forward)	1	n/a	20-30	2 RR	Moderate
Supine Hip Extension Push through heels and activate TVA to avoid lumbar hyperextension	1	n/a	20-30	2 RR	1-2-1
Arnie Press Don't allow pelvis to fall forward when fatigued	1	n/a	20-30	2 RR	Moderate
Overhand Pull-Downs Bring bar below chin but not below clavicle	1	90 sec	20-30	2 RR	Moderate

Exercises (circuit 2)	Sets	Rest	Reps	Intensity	Tempo/ Duration
Side Lunge Begin with non-dominant leg and alternate	1	n/a	20-30 each side, alternating	2 RR	Moderate
Unilateral Low Row Begin with non-dominant side	1	n/a	20-30 each	2 RR	Moderate

Exercises (circuit 2)	Sets	Rest	Reps	Intensity	Tempo/ Duration
Unilateral Supine Hip-Extension When unable to continue on one leg, use two legs for the remaining reps	1	n/a	20-30 each	2 RR	1-2-1
Med Ball Push-Ups Maintain **neutral spine**. Go to knees as necessary	1	n/a	20-30	2 RR	Moderate
Unilateral Cable Pulls Vary stance as proficiency allows	1	90 sec	20-30 each	2 RR	Moderate

Exercises (circuit 3—only when no DOMS)	Sets	Rest	Reps	Intensity	Tempo/ Duration
Dead Lift Push the ground away and maintain TVA activation	0-1	n/a	20-30	2 RR	Moderate
Bent-Over Row Maintain lordosis and HIGH elbows	0-1	n/a	20-30	2 RR	1-2-1
Unilateral Supine Hip Extension Knee Flexion When unable to continue with one leg, use two legs for the remaining reps	0-1	n/a	20-30 each	2 RR	1-2-1
Unilateral Cable Push Begin with non-dominant side and vary stance as proficiency allows	0-1	n/a	20-30 each	2 RR	Moderate

Exercises (circuit 3)	Sets	Rest	Reps	Intensity	Tempo/ Duration
Chin Ups (with assistance) Keep hips underneath shoulders (i.e., don't allow pelvis to sway forward)	0-1	90 sec	20-30	2 RR	Moderate

CORE Specific	Sets	Rest	Reps	Intensity	Tempo/ Duration
Alternating Superman on Ball Arm comes out at 45° from body, leading with the thumb	1	30 sec	8-12 each side	1 RR	Moderate with controlled PAUSE at top
Reverse Hyperextension on Ball Keep legs straight, extending from hips	1	45 sec	8-12	1 RR	Moderate with controlled PAUSE at top
Prone Cobra Don't look forward— keep head aligned with rest of spine	1	60 sec	1	1 RR	30-180 sec HOLD
Lower Abdominal #2A Only move leg in a R.O.M. which allows perfect form (i.e., back flat)	1	60 sec	8-12 each side	1 RR or 40mmHg + 30mmHg	Slow/ controlled
Oblique Raise Keep body one straight line from ankles to ears	1	60 sec	1	1 RR	20-30 sec HOLD
Stabilizer Use a dowel rod for cueing if unable to recognize what a neutral spine should feel like	1	n/a	1	1 RR	20-60 sec HOLD

NOTES FOR ALL WEIGHT-TRAINING PHASES:

An explanation of the specific column headings is warranted. Exercises, Sets, Rest, and Reps should all be pretty self-explanatory. Under the Intensity column, the notation 2 RR stands for 2 Repetition Reserve. This means that you should use a weight (i.e., intensity) that allows you to finish the prescribed number of repetitions and still have enough strength to do two more quality repetitions with good form. If you could do fifteen more reps, then the weight was too light. If you can't even finish the designated number of reps, then the weight was too heavy. Under the Tempo column, the speed of the lift is specified:

- Moderate is how most lifts are naturally performed and is considered the baseline speed.

- Slow is approximately half the pace of Moderate so the lift takes twice as long to perform.

- Fast is approximately twice the pace of Moderate so the lift takes half as long to perform.

- Explosive is the fastest pace possible for the weight of the lift.

- terms such as HOLD designate one repetition which is held statically for a period of time (i.e., 20-30s HOLD = a contraction/position held for twenty to thirty seconds).

- terms with numbers (i.e., 1-2-1) are written to indicate a specific lifting speed where the first number indicates the duration in seconds for the concentric portion of the lift. The second number is the pause, if any. And the third number is the duration in seconds for the eccentric portion of the lift.

ALWAYS include at least one warm-up set at 50-60% of the work weight to activate the musculature used with the pattern in which it will be exercised. This set does NOT count as one of the two to three work sets used during this phase. Once a specific body part is warm, additional warm up sets are not necessary. Thus, if you perform a lunge after having performed a squat, you don't need to perform a warm-up set of lunges since the legs are already warm. However, just because you have performed a pull exercise for the upper body doesn't mean you have warmed up the muscles of your upper body which perform pushing movements.

When exercising unilaterally, ALWAYS begin the movement with the **non-dominant** side. Non-dominance is determined by:

- Side preference (i.e., a right-handed athlete would begin movements of the upper body with his/her *left* hand)

- Side which is injured or inhibited (i.e., an athlete who is rehabbing his/her injured right knee would begin unilateral movements with the right leg *even if the athlete is right-side dominant*). Fatigue is cumulative. Thus, an athlete should perform unilateral movements on the weaker/injured/inhibited side first so that the athlete can allot more neural drive to the side which demands more attention before fatigue begins to degrade movement quality.

   *This is an excellent phase in which the athlete can take measures to balance the level of function in the body by performing extra sets or extra reps on the non-dominant side when exercising unilaterally.

BREATHING

Breathing is of critical importance to a successful strength-training program. Optimal breathing patterns will minimize the risk of injury while maximizing the benefit of the triathlete's time in the weight room. Specifically, inhalations should occur during movements where the body moves out of or away from the fetal position; while exhalations should be reserved for movements that move the body toward or into the fetal position. This is exactly how the body works. Try it: Take a big breath in and notice that you get taller as your spine elongates into extension. Now blow the air out of your lungs and feel how you get shorter as you literally compress into flexion. In a properly functioning body, inhaling is coupled with axial extension and exhaling is coupled with flexion of the axial skeleton. Lifting with proper breathing mechanics will help you be stronger during the lift.

The one exception to this rule is when lifting at intensities that necessitate holding one's breath. The body does this naturally as a way to stabilize the diaphragm so the muscles of the inner unit have a solid foundation from which to apply force and stabilize the axial skeleton. Failure to do so would send excessive loads through the spine, eventually resulting in injury. Thus, using a heavy back squat as an example, optimal breathing for a safe and successful lift would proceed in the following order:

1. INHALE to charge the thoracic cavity.

2. Gently draw in the belly button to activate the TVA.

3. Descend in a controlled manner with knees tracking over toes and your pressure through the heels.

4. Once at parallel or at the appropriate depth based on the ability to maintain a lumbar lordosis, begin the ascent. EXHALE through pursed lips after passing through the sticking point as you return to the start position.

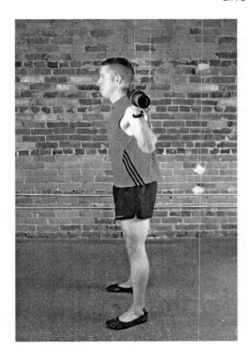 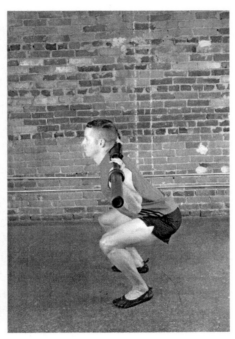

SQUAT

A more thorough discussion on the importance of proper breathing mechanics can be found in chapter three of the following section.

EXECUTION—How to implement all five of the training phases will be addressed in Chapter One of Section Four.

I advise athletes with a training age of *less than one year* to focus on the Anatomical Adaptation phase for a total of eight weeks before continuing on to the final two of the five weight-training phases. The Maximum Strength phase and the Power Complexity phase are best reserved for athletes with a training age of at least two years. Training age is defined as the number of years an athlete has been performing weights *without an extended break (one year or more) from training for injury or other reason(s)*. E.g., a twenty-five-year-old triathlete who performed strength training for four years in high school as a component of his or her swim training but only got back into the weight room at the age of twenty-four has a training age of one year.

CHAPTER 2:
The Maximum Strength Phase (MS)

I firmly believe in resistance training with heavy weights. So long as I taper

sufficiently before a race, I feel they improve my performance.

—Marianne Kriel, 1996 Olympic swimming medalist

We're triathletes, for crying out loud! What possible reason could we have for lifting so much freakin' weight? Heck, with the carbon-fiber bar tape you just bought, your bike only weighs 14.3 pounds! You can get it on the roof rack of your car without going anaerobic, so you're obviously strong enough.

Strength, as defined by Bompa in *Periodization: Theory and Methodology of Training*, is "the neuromuscular capability to overcome an external and internal resistance." The strength of an athlete is determined by how much work that athlete can perform. In triathlon, then, the competitor must be strong enough to complete the distance. So if you cross the finish line, is this strong enough?

No matter where you placed in your last tri, you covered the same distance as all the other competitors. You got the work done. As a matter of fact, since you all completed the same course, it could be said that you are all equally strong. But that would be inaccurate.

Let's say that you're a Clydesdale who always wins his category but just misses out on taking the overall title. So you cherrypick a small Olympic distance race in the middle of nowhere and peak for it like it's the World Championships. You've visualized this race a thousand times and already have a spot picked out for the overall trophy on your wall of fame. You're gonna rock!

And then I show up.

I live nowhere near the race venue. But I happen to be attending my grandmother's ninetieth birthday party and hear about this race at the last minute while stopping to use the bathroom at the local Waffle Hut which is sponsoring the event (I wouldn't eat there!). You see me in the transition area and immediately mark me as possible competition. After all, I have a carbon-fiber Cervelo and the absence of a mullet

115

makes me conspicuous among the rest of the field. But at a buck thirty, I'm not an impressive figure, so you're not terribly worried as we wade out into the water together.

And then I beat you.

Only by a second or two, but I beat you. You put a minute on me out of the water. Then I catch you on the bike, hammering back to transition to start the run with almost a two-minute advantage. Your long legs eat up most of my lead during the final leg, but, in the end, you run out of real estate and cross the finish a few steps behind me. You're bummed but console yourself with the knowledge that you made me work for the win, saying you simply lost to a stronger athlete.

How wrong you are.

You weigh 200 pounds. I weigh 130. We both covered the same distance. But you had to carry an additional 70 pounds over the course of the race. Technically, you did more work. Work is force applied over distance. It is the product of the amount of resistance overcome (200 pounds vs. 130 pounds) and the distance over which that resistance is moved (an Olympic distance triathlon). *You* are the stronger athlete. Strap a 70 pound weight to my body, and I would probably still be at the bottom of the lake somewhere.

I know, I'm not making much of a case for strength training here. I mean, if it's not the strongest athlete who wins, why lift weights, right? If you're thinking like that, I can tell you've skipped the first several chapters of this book. There's a multitude of reasons, but let's look at strength and its critical role in the performance of a triathlon.

If we change some of the parameters of the imaginary race cited above, it may provide you with a clearer understanding of the importance of strength in our sport. Let's say I let myself go a bit during the off season—to the tune of seventy pounds. I win a year's supply of Breyer's Mint Chocolate Chip and decide I'm going to test out the Ullrich Theory of Performance Enhancement. We both show up on the starting line, but this time I'm 200 pounds, same as you. You win the race walking away, with a personal best of two hours even. I score a different type of PR—four hours. You probably could've lapped me if you'd run the course a second time. Obviously you're the stronger athlete now, right?

Wrong again.

Once more, we both completed the same distance. Yet now we weigh the same.

We both did the same work. It doesn't matter if I took twice as long as you to cover the distance, as time is a variable which does not enter into the strength equation. Time is important in the equation for *power*. By the strictest definition of strength, we are both equal despite the fact you had enough time to shower, eat, and overhaul your bottom bracket before I crossed the finish line.

Why then, are we wasting our time on strength development? Why not just skip to power training (no pun intended) if that's what's really going to determine who finishes a particular race in first place?

Power is how much work is done per unit of time or, expressed as an equation:

$$\textbf{POWER} = \frac{\textit{FORCE (i.e., strength)} \times \textit{DISTANCE}}{\textbf{TIME}}$$

The reason triathletes must first focus on strength is because this biomotor ability is a crucial component in the optimal development of power. Tudor Bompa, in his groundbreaking book *Periodization: Theory and Methodology of Training*, agrees. Strength development, he says, "should be the prime concern of anyone who attempts to improve an athlete's performance." Its importance is again highlighted on a page from *Advanced Program Design*, which states, "When strength or any of its derivatives are the primary deficit, efforts should focus primarily on its development first." Thus, to maximize power development, we must either maximize strength or maximize speed, or, with a good training program, maximize both.

Maximum Strength is the highest force that can be performed by the neuromuscular system during a maximum voluntary contraction.

$$\textbf{FORCE} = \textbf{MASS} \times \textit{ACCELERATION} \ (F = M \times A)$$

So to increase the force produced, we can increase the resistance (M) or the speed at which the resistance is moved (A). Yet increasing movement speed is not as effective in the development of maximum strength as increasing the weight of the resistance, due primarily to the role momentum plays in the lift.

Momentum is mass in motion. For those of you who fell asleep in physics class, I'll keep this simple. The more mass or velocity an object has, the more momentum that object will possess. That's one reason why you see some people swinging their free weights around and rushing through a set of twelve like their lives depend on it. The only newton they've ever heard of is a cookie. But they innately know that once they start their hundred-pound bicep curl with their back and knees, their arms can go along for the ride. Momentum is their ego's best friend.

Maximal tension on a muscle, which is critical for maximal strength development, is only increased during the initial acceleration of the load. After that, momentum takes over and effectively reduces the tensile loading of the muscle. But if you use a sufficiently heavy weight, the speed at which the weight is lifted will be limited. Thus, the contribution of momentum to the lift will be minimized, as well.

This is not to say that you should not *try* to accelerate the load as quickly as possible. To quote Chek again, "The closer a given load is moved to maximum velocity the greater the intensity and the greater the training effect on a neuromuscular basis." The neuromuscular benefits to which Chek refers are:

increased neural drive to the muscle
increased synchronization of motor units
increased activation of the contractile apparatus
decreased inhibition of the protective mechanisms of the muscle
(Golgi tendon organ).

Basically, you're making the muscle smarter when you challenge it with a sufficient resistance, literally putting brains behind that brawn. And a smart, functional muscle is a strong muscle.

Strength is, ironically, often an endurance athlete's biggest weakness. But the intelligent triathlete quickly learns to apply this one golden rule: Train your weaknesses and race your strengths. And I must warn you, this phase is not easy. The absolute antithesis of endurance training, the Maximum Strength phase, is going to challenge you in ways you might have never before experienced. You may encounter soreness which will leave you temporarily unable to sit down on the toilet seat. Your legs will probably bitch at you for the first twenty-nine minutes of a half-hour run. But the biggest obstacle you'll face is the misinformation with which you've been programmed about lifting heavy weights.

How heavy am I talking about??? Heavy! At least 85% of your one-rep max. This equates to one to six reps. And, no, you're not going to end up looking like Conan the Barbarian. I tell my female clients that, unless they're shaving their faces twice a day, they probably don't have enough of the right hormones in their body to get big. And this is true for my male clients, as well. It's probably one reason why they were drawn to a sport like triathlon in the first place. Yet sometimes this fear cannot be vanquished until I quote Tudor Bompa, who holds that "maximum strength gains… are up to three times greater than the proportional gain in muscle hypertrophy" when employing maximal loads. Roughly translated for the physiologically illiterate— lift correctly and you'll get strong rather than big.

These strength gains come, in large part, from an increase in **motor unit** activation. While novice athletes generally recruit around 60% of their available motor units, a properly designed strength-training program can increase this number up to 85%. And which carriage do you think can go farther and faster—the one pulled by sixty horses or the one pulled by eight-five?

Most of this difference results from a greater number of fast-twitch motor units doing some of the work. According to the size principle, in muscles with a combination of type I and type II fibers, motor units are recruited according to their size with the smaller, slow-twitch fibers (type I) preferentially recruited over the more powerful fast-twitch fibers (type II). Athletes who do not often train at intensities high enough to recruit the fast-twitch muscle fibers regularly have allowed these potential workhorses to wander out to pasture and become lazy. And in the rare times that they are called upon to help the athlete during a race, they often can't remember in which direction the barn is located. This leads to an uncoordinated and inefficient muscular response and an athlete unable to reach his or her potential.

Another determining factor in the successful acquisition of strength which takes place at the neural level is how quickly the motor units fire. Norman Jones, in his book entitled *Human Muscle Power*, refers to a number of studies that show high-intensity strength training improves the firing rate of motor units. Tudor Bompa again confirms these findings:

> Maximum strength is also a function of the intensity of an impulse, which
>
> dictates the number of motor units involved, and its frequency. According
>
> to Zatzyorski (1968), the number of impulses per second may elevate from
>
> five or six at rest, up to fifty, lifting a maximum load.

So, I ask you. As the owner of a business, which would you prefer? A training program which teaches your employees to do five or six tasks a second or one which can teach them to do fifty? It's your body. And that's your business. But personally, I'd choose the one which destines my company to success. Your business just can't survive in a competitive environment otherwise. Similarly, you simply will not win in the world of triathlon if your body is still functioning like a mom-n-pop dime store.

REST PERIODS

All these neural adaptations will only take place if you allow the central nervous system to recover appropriately. Too short a rest interval and you begin to tap into alternate energy systems—from the phosphagen system, to the glycolytic, and then into the oxidative (aerobic) energy system. This is not to suggest, as many

119

people erroneously believe, that energy during activity is supplied by only one system to the exclusion of the other two. In fact, all three are active at any give time. However, intensity of the activity and, to a large extent, the duration of the activity will determine the extent to which each system is used.

Cardio manufacturers have popularized the idea that working out at a specific level will allow the body to burn more fat. And in our fat-phobic society, this belief has led to a gym industry which caters to cardio. Walk into any fitness facility in the US and you'll see thousands of dollars' worth of treadmills, ellipticals, stairmasters, and bikes. Attached to each will be a sign-up list to keep the waiting masses in order until they can enter "the fat-burning zone."

And while it may be true that exercising in this zone utilizes a greater percentage of calories from fat, the numbers can be misleading. Let's take a 150-pound male who, when running at six miles per hour, is comfortably in the famous fat-burning zone. Burning approximately six hundred calories during the course of his one hour workout, his contribution from fat will be around 50% or three hundred calories. Now take this same guy and have him run eight miles per hour. He burns approximately eight hundred calories, but only 40% came from fat. Yet, 40% of eight hundred is 320. The total contribution from his fat stores is actually higher despite working above the so-called fat-burning zone. And he burns more calories in the same amount of time.

*Additionally, the calories expended after cessation of exercise, referred to as "excess post-exercise oxygen consumption" or **EPOC**, will keep his metabolism well above its normal resting rate for minutes or even hours once his run is finished. After all, it requires energy to remove lactate, replenish oxygen stores, resynthesize the ATP-PC system, and to bring the body's systems back to pre-exercise levels in general. And while all of these factors can be affected not only by the duration and intensity of the exercise but also by gender, training status, and even timing of the exercise session, one truth is without debate: When measured strictly by percentage of contribution, the best fat-burning activity is simply going to sleep. And that's one thing the cardio manufacturers can't sell you. No, the drug companies have exclusive rights to that...*

Energy production by aerobic metabolism is an unwanted result of insufficient rest during this phase. As Chek points out in *Program Design*, "inadequate rest will result in forced recruitment of IIa and eventually type I fibers. This will significantly effect (sic) speed of movement, strength, and muscle tension." In addition, increased recruitment of the oxidative system promotes the release of **cortisol** and other **glucocorticoids** which are antagonistic to maximal strength development (for a more detailed explanation of glucocorticoids, please refer to Chapter Two of Section Four below).

Motor learning is also adversely affected by short rest intervals as fatigue detracts from the performance of the athlete. Bompa states that inadequate rest "between two sets of maximum contraction (is) not sufficient to relax and regenerate the neuromuscular system to achieve high activation in the subsequent set." The neural fatigue the athlete then experiences retards motor skill development resulting in the athlete being "programmed" with *slow*, less powerful movements.

So you gotta rest! But not too much, as an excessive rest interval has its own detriments, too. Your neurological system suffers from a bit of ADD. If the athlete rests too long between sets, his or her nervous system loses its excitation and gets bored, creating an unfriendly atmosphere for learning and performance. Combined with a loss of body temperature, this can result in injury to the athlete as the warm up has effectively been lost.

Thus, in the Maximum Strength phase, it is generally agreed that the fine line between too much rest and too little recovery is three to five minutes. That's a lot of time between sets, I know. So I'll normally fill that time with dynamic stretching or, when I'm in my studio, listening to lectures on nutrition or kinesiology or maybe quantum physics. I may even write poetry or something to get me out of my left brain for a bit—that's good for mental recovery. Yet sometimes all I want to do is sit and chill for a few minutes as I recover from the effort of the previous set.

One last recommendation before I describe the specifics of the Maximum Strength phase: I try to make each successive set of the exercises in **BOLD** a bit heavier than the one before it. Just like when I do intervals, making each effort faster than the one before it, adding weight each set teaches my body to perform at a continuously high level while in a fatigued state. This is critical as the person who wins the race, especially at Ironman distance, is often the athlete who slows down the least.

Maximum Strength Phase Details

- Station Training—Finish all sets of the exercise before going on to the next movement except as noted with supersets

- 85-95% of 1RM

- 3-5 sets for exercises in **BOLD**

- 3-5 minutes between sets for exercises in **BOLD**

- 3-6 reps for exercises in **BOLD**—try to lift the weight EXPLOSIVELY or as QUICKLY as possible. The negative (eccentric motion) should be slow and controlled

- 2-3 days a week on non-consecutive days

- Use every third or fourth week as a recovery week by following the guidelines in Chapter One of Section Four below

- Four weeks for experienced lifters before changing phases; six weeks for novice lifters

- ALWAYS warm up to your work weight with 1-3 progressively heavier sets (i.e., 5 sets of 150 lbs. max with warm-up sets of 50 lbs. and then 90 lbs.)

- Exercises not in bold are 3 sets of 20-30 reps with 1 minute rest in between each

- Abs and back are either timed, if static contractions, or 8-20 reps for 3 sets

- Follow the order of exercises

- 1 hour approximate workout time

  1. **Squat Pattern Exercise or Dead Lift**—Foot position should replicate pedal position! Choose one exercise and continue training that movement for at least three weeks.

  2. **Seated Swiss Ball Row/Pull-Ups**—Alternate from week to week. Hand position should replicate swim or handlebar position.

  3. Push Pattern Exercise—Change exercises each week. **Superset** with exercise #4 below.

  4. Bend Pattern Exercise superset with exercise #3 above.

  5. Abdominal superset with #6 below.

  6. Back Extension (found in the BEND PATTERN section)—Performed on unstable surface (i.e., a Swiss Ball). Superset with #5 above.

Exercises	Sets	Rest	Reps	Intensity	Tempo/ Duration
High Step Up Begin with NON-dominant side.	3-5	3-5 min	2-6 each side	2RR	Fast intent on Positive
Pull Ups Position hands swim-width apart	3-4	3-5 min	2-6	1 RR	Fast intent on Positive
Kneeling-on-Physio-Ball Arnie Press (Alternating) Begin with NON-dominant side and superset with Bent-Over Row below.	2-3	n/a	20-30 each side, alternating	1 RR	Moderate
Bent-Over Row Maintain lordosis and HIGH elbows.	2-3	45 sec	20-30	1 RR	1-3-1
Lower Abdominal #1 Superset with Alternating Superman below. Do one set of this exercise DAILY	1-3	n/a	12-20	1 RR or 40mmHg + 30mmHg	Slow/ controlled
Alternating Superman Arm out at 45°, leading with thumb.	2-3	45 sec	12-20 each side, alternating	1 RR	1-3-1

CHAPTER 3:
The Power Complexity Phase (PC)

When all other factors are equal, power is the deciding factor between winning and losing.

—Patrick O'Shea

In the previous chapter, I described two theoretical scenarios comparing two triathletes to demonstrate why maximum strength, while a foundation of optimal physical performance, cannot be the sole focus of a successful weight-training program for multisport. Another real-life example of why we cannot spend all of our time training at the slow speeds inherent to the MS phase can probably be found at your next triathlon: the big, muscular competitor who finishes an hour behind you.

When you first saw this guy at the start line, you may have thought he was going to rip your legs off. You may have even felt sorry for his bike. But his placement behind you in the overall, assuming he didn't take a wrong turn out on the course somewhere, is probably best explained by the force-velocity curve seen in the FIGURE 1 to the right.

Figure1. The Force-Velocity Curve

Simply put, to the degree one moves farther along the vertical axis of force (i.e., strength), velocity will diminish. The movements which occur during the Maximum Strength phase of weights require a lot of force but occur at a low velocity. It takes time to produce maximal force—400 milliseconds to be exact (in contrast, the amount of time a sprinter's foot will be in contact with the ground during each stride is approximately 100 milliseconds). Thus, as one moves closer to his/her **One-Rep Max**, the speed at which the resistance is moved will decrease until the point at which movement ceases: The person cannot produce any more force. At maximal force generation, there is no velocity. The contraction of the muscle is isometric.

So, yes, that hulk that looked great in his trisuit but still wasn't back to T2 when you crossed the finish line is strong. In fact, he's probably somewhere near the top of the Force axis in the figure above. But his corresponding placement on the Velocity axis (horizontal line) is found on the far left of the diagram. He has no speed. Force and velocity are inversely proportional. As one goes up, the other goes down.

This begs for the question then: Why be strong at slow speeds when triathlon involves higher-velocity movements? The SAID principle discussed in Chapter 5 of the preceding section illustrates the point. In simple terms, this concept holds that the targeted system gets better at *exactly* what it does. Practice the piano, get better at playing the piano. Perform a skill, get better at that particular skill. Train slow. Be slow.

And that's the reason why weight training for the intelligent triathlete doesn't end with the Maximum Strength phase. Just like in triathlon, there's another leg to complete before the finish line is reached. Force has been developed—maybe even maximized with hard work. And that work has established the foundation on which movement speed can reach its potential during the Power Complexity phase. Stop now and you'll be that triathlete whom nobody wants to arm wrestle but everyone can't wait to race—strong, but with no speed.

PLYOMETRICS

Plyometrics are movements that teach the body to recruit the maximal amount of force in the shortest amount of time. Sounds like the definition of power, right? Used appropriately, plyometric training is the key to transferring the strength built in the weight room to speed in the competitive environment. They will help move the force-velocity curve up and to the right. Properly implemented into your training program, plyometrics will make you faster.

Try this experiment. Stand next to a wall with your hands above your head and jump as high as you can. Note how high you got. Now move away from the wall before you do a second attempt. This time, take a couple of steps toward the wall and then quickly drop into a partial squat before exploding up off the ground. You jumped higher this time, didn't you? What you just experienced is a live demonstration of the **Stretch-Shortening Cycle**—the underlying principle of plyometric training.

One of the mechanisms by which the body conserves energy to move more efficiently, the stretch-shortening cycle is an active stretching of a muscle under load **(eccentric contraction)** followed by an immediate shortening of the muscle **(concentric contraction)**. The time between the start of eccentric movement and the start of the concentric movement is called the **amortization phase**. During this period, elastic energy is stored in the muscle tendon unit. If the transition between eccentric loading and concentric movement takes too long, this elastic energy is dissipated as heat. However, if this transition occurs rapidly enough, the stored energy is utilized to make the subsequent movement not only more efficient but more powerful as well.

The last time you had a physical, you probably had the doctor tap your patella tendon with a small rubber hammer. And if he hit the right spot the right way, you had an involuntary contraction which would've made him a soprano if he had been standing in front of you. You had no control over your leg, so you'd get to take no credit for his new singing career. That was the stretch reflex, or myotatic reflex, in action. And that's the basis of plyometrics.

Unlike voluntary actions, which originate in the brain and travel down the spinal cord to the specific body part(s), the impulse during a myotatic reflex travels from the muscle spindle involved in an action to the spinal cord and back. It doesn't have to go all the way to the brain, so the reaction is much quicker—one to two milliseconds on average. The whole process is a protective measure to keep the muscles from tearing. When the muscle spindle is rapidly stretched, an impulse is almost instantaneously received to contract quickly so the muscle is not pulled beyond its normal, healthy range of motion.

So when the doctor tapped the hammer just below your knee, your patella tendon was stretched and your quadriceps contracted. Had he gently pushed on the tendon, however, your leg would've just sat there as it's the rate and force at which the spindle is stretched which dictates how powerfully the muscle contracts. It should come as no surprise then that these two specific components, rate (i.e., velocity) and force, will be crucial in the development of your power when using plyometrics during this phase of weight training.

127

PLYOMETRIC PRECAUTIONS and PROCEDURES

How much weight could you squat when you were in elementary school? Any idea? Well, what about your bench—how much could you bench press? The National Strength and Conditioning Association (NSCA) holds that a minimum level of strength should be reached before including plyometrics in a training program. For lower-body movements, the NSCA recommends that a person be able to squat 1.5 to 2.5 times his/her body weight. For upper-body movements, being able to bench press 1 to 1.5 times body weight is considered the minimum strength requirement. Yet literally thousands of kids play hopscotch—basically a plyometric workout—every day at school. And many of them are playing freeze tag or kick ball or capture the flag or any of a number of games where the child runs, which, in essence, is plyometric training. Who cleared them to do that? Where are the waivers they signed?

I'm not downplaying the importance of preparation and proper progression in a training program. In fact, the premise of this book is founded on how the body works and adapts when exposed to specific stimuli which, with critical analysis and simple periodization techniques, can be manipulated to create the desired outcome. For you, the triathlete, that outcome means swimming, cycling, and running to the limit of your genetic potential—an achievement about which few of us can boast because we seem stuck at a certain speed or, worse yet, stuck on the sidelines with a nagging injury.

If you've followed the principles outlined in this book, then you've developed the necessary flexibility and stability which are the essential foundation upon which strength is built. You have then maximized force production with functional exercises specific to your training needs and abilities. Now you are finally ready to turn that strength into power—power which will make you not only faster and more resilient. It will make that jump to the top of the podium easier, too.

In the Power Complexity phase of weights, plyometric training is coupled with strength training by performing a specific lift followed immediately by an explosive activity which closely resembles the previous movement. For example, a set of Exploding Harvards would be performed directly following a set of Step Ups. This combination more effectively targets the Type IIb muscle fibers, also referred to as the fast glycolytic fibers—the ones responsible for explosive force production.

The idea is simple: The heavy resistance ramps up the recruitment of the Type IIb fibers so that more of these powerhouses are available to perform the explosive movement which follows. Actually getting these fibers to work is a bit more difficult, however. Gently hopping around after doing a lift isn't going to cut it. The fast glycolytic fibers are powerful, but they're slow to get their ass in gear. So, instead of contributing, the Type IIb fibers will allow first the Type I and then the Type IIa fibers to do all the work if your intensity is lacking. Only when the task performed requires maximal force will the Type IIb fibers step up.

This means that recovery, just like in the Maximal Strength phase, will be of the utmost importance when training for power. Not only will the Type IIb fibers remain dormant until you truly need them; they'll also fatigue easily and require more time to rest before they're ready to go again. They are low in both mitochondrial and capillary density and will not recuperate as quickly or as efficiently as Type I or Type IIa fibers will. Thus, the rest between sets during the Power Complexity phase will be three to five minutes so that the succeeding set will suffer no drop-off in intensity.

Power Complexity Phase Details

- 70-85% of 1 RM

- 3-5 sets for exercises in **BOLD**

- 3-5 minutes between sets for exercises in **BOLD**

- 3-6 reps for exercises in **BOLD**, performing the concentric as fast as possible

   IMMEDIATELY followed by a Plyometric Drill for 6 reps or 8 seconds, whichever comes first

   NOTE: the prescribed intensity for the weight training is less than the repetition range prescribed—you should have more reps "left in the tank."

- 2 days a week on non-consecutive days

- 72 hours between workouts

- Use every third or fourth week as a recovery week by following the guidelines in Chapter One of Section Four below

- Four weeks for experienced lifters before changing phases; six weeks for novice lifters

- Contacts for NOVICE: 60-100

- Contacts for INTERMEDIATE: 100-150

- Contacts for ADVANCED: 150-200

   A **contact** is any time the feet touch the ground or the hands touch the ground/training implement during a Plyometric Drill.

- Follow the order of the exercises

- 51 minutes approximate workout time

   1. **Squat/Lunge Pattern Exercise or Dead Lift**—Foot position should replicate pedal position! Choose one exercise and continue training that movement for two weeks. Superset with exercise #2 below.

   2. **Plyometric Drill** most closely resembling the movement above. Superset with exercise #1 above.

   3. **Push Pattern Exercise**—change exercises each week. Superset with exercise # 4 below.

129

4. **Plyometric Drill** most closely resembling the movement above. Superset with exercise #3 above.

5. Pull Pattern Exercise.

6. Abdominal.

7. Back Extension (found in the BEND PATTERN section)—performed on unstable surface (i.e., a Swiss Ball).

Example Plyometric Drills

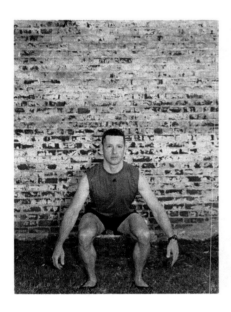 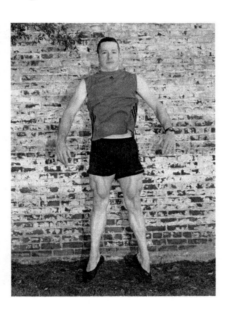

JUMPS AFTER SQUATS

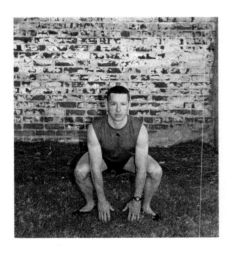 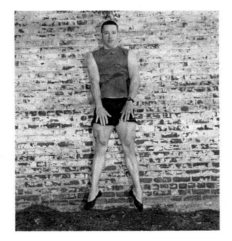

FROG JUMPS AFTER DEAD LIFTS

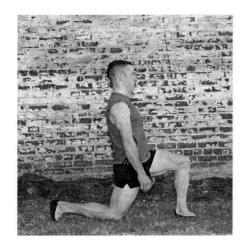 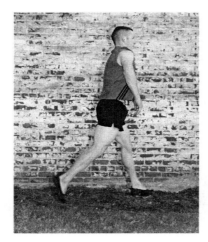 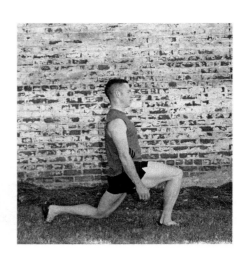

LUNGE HOPS AFTER LUNGES

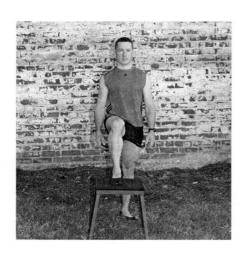 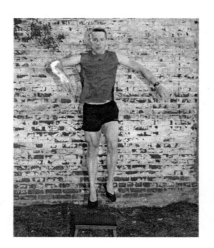 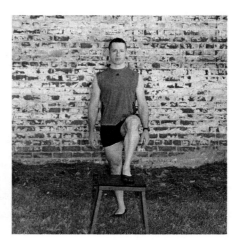

EXPLODING HARVARDS AFTER STEP UPS

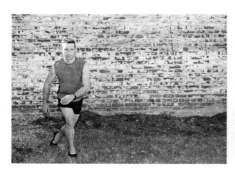 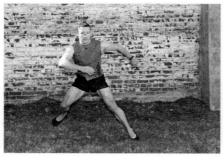 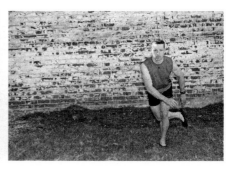

SLALOM HOPS AFTER SIDE LUNGES

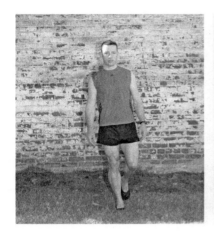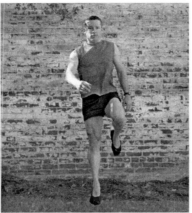

UNI HOPS AFTER UNILATERAL SQUATS

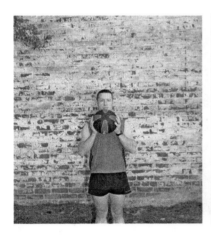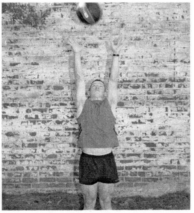

MED BALL OVERHEAD THROWS AFTER ARNIE PRESS

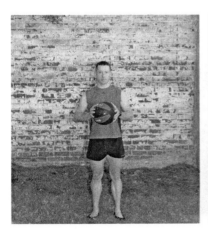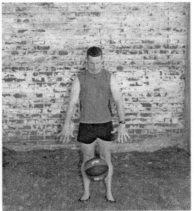

MED BALL TRICEP THROWS AFTER DECLINE PUSH UP

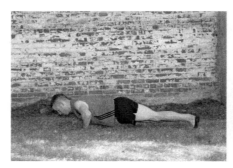
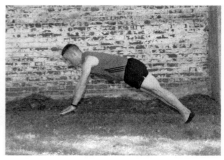

PLYO PUSH UPS AFTER PUSH UPS

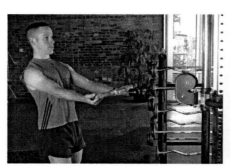
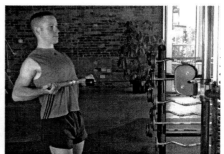

EXPLOSIVE ROWS AFTER ROWS

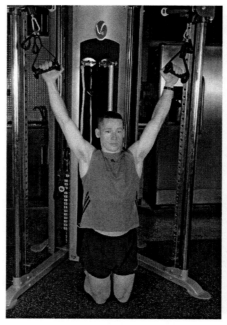
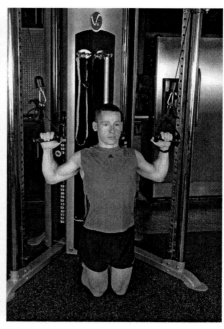

EXPLOSIVE PULL DOWNS AFTER PULL UPS

Exercises	Sets	Rest	Reps	Intensity	Tempo/ Duration
Dead Lifts Push the ground away. Superset with Frog Jumps below.	3-5	n/a	3-6	70-85% 1 RM	Fast intent on Positive
Frog Jumps Absorb landing and immediately explode up at maximal intensity.	3-5	3-5 min	6 reps or 8s worth, whichever is less	1 RR	Explosive
Push-Ups Feet/Foot on Swiss Ball Insure neutral spinal alignment Superset with Med-Ball Overhead Throws below.	2-3	n/a	4-6 each side, alternating	1 RR	1-2-1
Med-Ball Overhead Throws Absorb weight of med ball during the catching phase and then immediately throw ball away from body at maximal intensity.	2-3	3-4 mins	6 reps or 8s worth, whichever is less	1 RR	Explosive
Suspended Row Keep elbows HIGH and maintain neutral spine.	2-3	45 sec	20-30	1 RR	1-2-1
Forward Ball Roll Do this on one leg as proficiency allows.	2-3	60 sec	8-12	1 RR	1-3-1
Twisting Back Extension on Ball Maintain TVA activation.	2-3	30 sec	8-20 each side, alternating	1 RR	Moderate to fast

CHAPTER 4:
The Strength Maintenance Phase (SM)

As the season nears and the triathlete begins to spend more time in the pool and on the road, the temptation to skimp on weight training is magnified by key races which loom on the horizon. Luckily, the volume required to maintain strength is less than that required to build it. But it must be maintained! Failure to do so will often result in performance decline as strength levels deteriorate. And lots of endurance training actually increases this insult. The capacity of the triathlete's neuromuscular system to generate force rapidly becomes compromised as the season progresses if weight training is phased out of the training program.

Explanations differ, but the commonly accepted theory behind this deleterious decline in strength is altered testosterone-to-cortisol ratios, which leave the body in a **catabolic** state. The importance of these hormones is discussed in greater detail in Section Four. But for now, let's just say that an imbalance between the catabolic and **anabolic** systems is a state you want to avoid for extended periods of time.

137

In simple terms, the catabolic system breaks down the body, while the anabolic system is responsible for repair. In regards to training, a stimulus is provided which first causes a decline in fitness. If followed by an appropriate amount of rest positioned at the right time in the athlete's program, the body's anabolic system kicks in, allowing for what is termed **supercompensation**—the athlete becomes stronger, faster, and better able to withstand future training at a level more intense and/or of greater volume than was previously tolerated. See the figure below.

If the athlete continues to train and ignores the body's need to balance the catabolic stimulus of training with the proper anabolic stimuli including rest, the eventual outcome can be catastrophic. I have a client who exemplifies this exact scenario. A world-class swimmer, she came to me in a state of true adrenal exhaustion. She had spent the last several months sleeping as many as fifteen

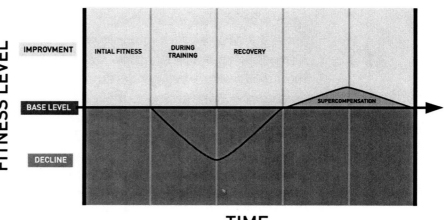

SUPERCOMPENSATION

hours a day while still waking up completely wiped out and unable to train. When asked, she admitted she hadn't had a period in many years. In addition to a diet consisting primarily of powerbars and synthetic crap void of any nutrition or life-giving properties, her recent athletic history had very few days of rest anywhere in the program. She literally was swimming on fumes. And she almost came to me too late. If you're interested, the details of her road to recovery can be found in the following section.

The Tour de France is another example of this scenario in action. During the course of three weeks, cyclists race over 2000 miles and place enormous demands on all the systems of the body. In fact, it's often said that the Tour takes four years off your life every time you do it. I don't know if that's true, but I do know one thing. Every cyclist who finishes a Grand Tour is slower, weaker, and less healthy than they were before the race. In fact, though the cyclists will often lose weight by the final stage into Paris, they actually gain body fat. That's right. The Tour de France makes them fat. They may be lighter when they race those final kilometers along the Champs-Elysees, but it's because they have less muscle mass.

In an effort to meet the excessive fueling requirements of such a long event, the body must catabolize muscle along with any other available protein source. Essential body organs, antibodies needed to fight infection, even simple enzymes are not spared as the body is convinced its survival is threatened. All of these adverse health reactions result in a slower cyclist, too. The winner of the Tour each year isn't necessarily the fastest cyclist in the peloton. He's the one who slowed down the least. Sounds kinda like the winner of the Ironman…

An additional consequence resulting from cessation of strength training is that the athlete's risk of injury increases. Compared to swimming, cycling, or even running, weight training carries the greatest osteogenic effect, increasing bone strength and bone-mineral content and thereby reducing the incidence of stress fractures. The resiliency of the body's connective tissue is also enhanced, with tendons and ligaments of resistance-trained athletes exhibiting greater size and strength than those not involved in weight training. Finally, muscle imbalances inherent to triathlon as mentioned earlier in this book can be addressed by focusing on the neglected musculature or devoting more time to strength development on the non-dominant/weaker side. This is critical to the triathlete's orthopedic integrity—the body doesn't mind weakness or tightness so much as a specific imbalance. Because with the imbalance comes compensations. And with the compensations come injuries.

The Strength Maintenance phase includes coordination drills specific to running. Placed immediately following the lower-body movement performed, the purpose of these drills is to help transfer the strength being maintained in the weight room to use during the competitive season. They also teach important concepts like ground-reaction time and proper landing mechanics. Of course, the Power Complexity phase helps accomplish these same goals with plyometric training. But the modest loads associated with the ladder and run drills (which are essentially plyometrics) of this phase allow for increased recuperation during what is likely a higher volume and intensity of run training for the athlete at this time of year. Additionally, rest intervals are kept at durations sufficient for ample recovery of both the muscular and nervous systems so that fatigue does not inhibit optimal programming of the athlete.

Strength Maintenance Phase Details

- 70-85% 1RM

- 2-3 sets (2 sets closer to competition and NO LEGS 10-14 days prior to GOAL EVENT and NO ARMS 7-10 days prior to GOAL EVENT). Drill and Core work can continue at intensities/volume which do not elicit delayed-onset muscle soreness (DOMS)

- 2-3 minutes between sets

- 6-12 reps

- Once every fourteen days, alternating with PPC phase (i.e., one week of SM followed by one week of PPC)

- Follow the order of the exercises

- 30 minutes approximate workout time

    1. **Lunge Pattern Exercise or Step Up**—Foot position should replicate pedal position! Choose one exercise and continue training that movement for 1 week, switching to a new movement the following week. Superset with exercise #2 below.

    2. **Running Drill or Ladder Drill for 8s.** Superset with exercise #1 above.

    3. **Push Pattern Exercise**—Change exercises each week. Superset with exercise # 4 below.

    4. Pull Pattern Exercise working in the same plane of motion as the movement above (i.e., a horizontal push is followed by a horizontal pull). Superset with exercise #3 above.

    5. Abdominal.

    6. Back-Extension (found in the BEND PATTERN section).

139

Example Run Drills

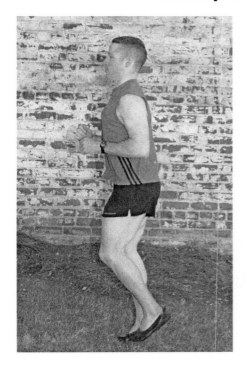 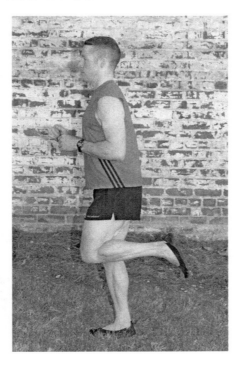

BUTT KICKS

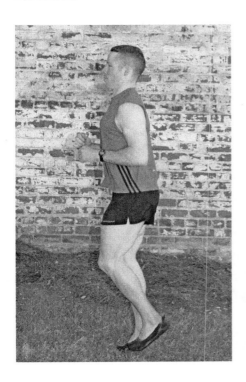 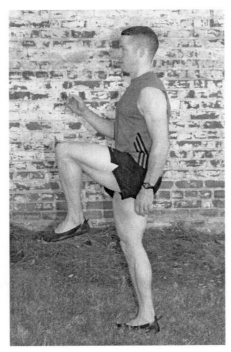

HIGH KNEES

Example Run Drills

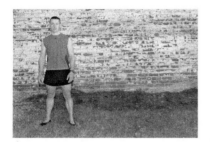

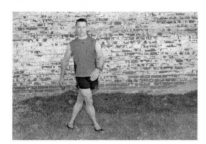

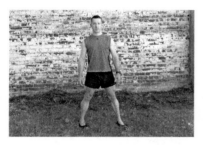

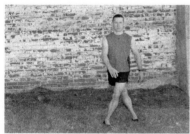

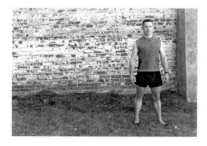

CARIOCA

SKIPPING

Example Ladder Drills

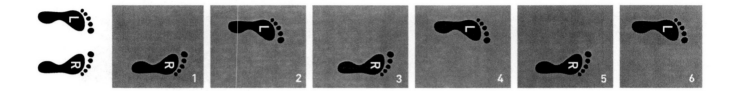

1 FOOT IN FORWARD

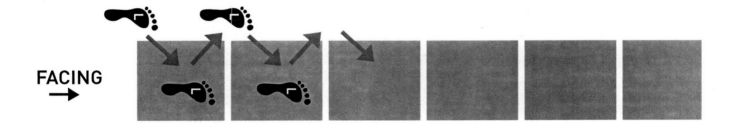

FACING

SINGLE LEG LATERAL HOPS

Example Ladder Drills

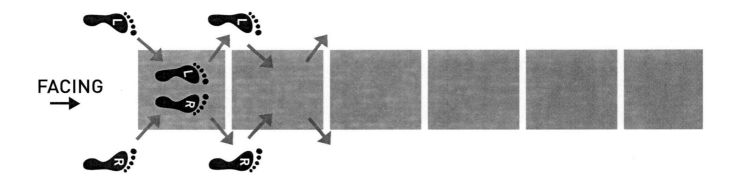

FACING

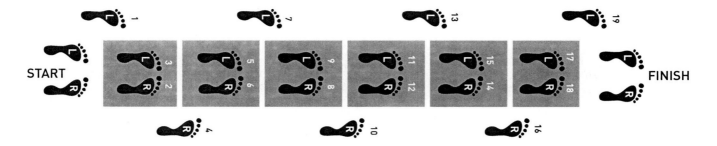

START

FINISH

Exercises	Sets	Rest	Reps	Intensity	Tempo/Duration
Step Up Bicep Curl Begin with non-dominant leg and curl opposite arm. Superset with Butt Kicks below.	2-3	n/a	6-8 each side, alternating	70-85% 1 RM	Fast intent on Positive
Butt Kicks Fast feet! Pretend the ground is HOT!	2-3	2-3 min	8s worth	1 RR	Explosive
T Push Ups Insure neutral spinal alignment. Superset with High Row with Rotation below.	2-3	n/a	4-6 each side, alternating	1 RR	Explosive with pause at end R.O.M.
High Row with Rotation Rotate then pull and keep elbows HIGH with palms facing down.	2-3	2-3 mins	10-12 each side, alternating	1 RR	Fast
Drop and Recover Use whole body, including legs.	2-3	45 sec	8-12 each side, alternating	1 RR	0-2-0
Alternating Superman (with Dumb Bells in Hands) Keep chin tucked and inhale into extension	2-3	45 sec	8-12	1 RR	1-3-1

CHAPTER 5:

Prehab and Postural Correction Phase (PPC)

Muscle imbalance may also result from occupational or recreational activities in which there is a persistent use of certain muscles without adequate exercise of opposing muscles. Imbalance that affects body alignment is an important factor in many painful postural conditions.

—Florence Kendall

The body always gravitates toward a position of strength. You're strong in the water, on the bike, and (if you're lucky) in your running shoes, too. And though you have been working out with renewed postural awareness, a well-designed weight program needs a period focusing on countering the influence a high volume of endurance training will have on your body. So, this final phase of strength training, called the Prehab and Postural Correction phase, will concentrate specifically on reversing the postural aberrations which are incurred with triathlon training and racing. Additionally, specific exercises will be included which will target key areas where pain often manifests due to local weakness.

So what are the weak links of a triathlete in the middle of the season? Well, the one who has been diligent with strength training throughout the year will have fewer than the competition. Resiliency built with proper resistance training will help an athlete endure the demands of triathlon better than his counterpart. Nonetheless, there are areas of weakness inherent to all three disciplines in a triathlon. In swimming, it's typically the shoulders. The lower back is the most common source of dysfunction for the cyclist. And the Achilles heel of runners is... well... the Achilles. In addition, the two areas which work with the ankle to make up the lower-body triple extensors—the knee and the hip—are sites where the triathlete's body will commonly break down.

Swimming and the Shoulder

The shoulder (glenohumeral joint) is the most mobile joint in the body. Yet a general principle regarding joint movement holds that flexibility and stability are inversely proportional. As one goes up, the other goes down. Thus the shoulder, capable

147

of working through an extraordinary range of motion and in all three planes of movement, is also extremely unstable. This instability often leads to fatigue of the dynamic stabilizers of the shoulder: the deltoid, the scapulae stabilizing muscles, and the infamous rotator cuff.

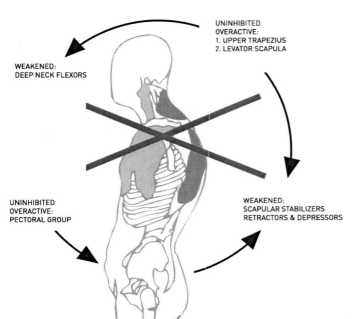

UNINHIBITED
OVERACTIVE:
1. UPPER TRAPEZIUS
2. LEVATOR SCAPULA

WEAKENED:
DEEP NECK FLEXORS

UNINHIBITED
OVERACTIVE:
PECTORAL GROUP

WEAKENED:
SCAPULAR STABILIZERS
RETRACTORS & DEPRESSORS

Consisting of four small muscles—infraspinatus, supraspinatus, subscapularis, and teres minor—the rotator cuff has a bad reputation among triathletes, because it's often the source of shoulder dysfunction which presents as pain during the swim. But the real blame for any of the syndromes which often cause pain when swimming lies, ironically, on the triathlete's shoulders. Swimming, cycling, and to some extent running all disproportionately develop the internal shoulder rotators in relation to the external shoulder rotators. Sitting and working in front of computers with faulty posture furthers this imbalance, leading to what's called an **Upper Cross Syndrome**.

With the Upper Cross Syndrome, the pectorals and the other internal shoulder rotators are short and tight while their respective antagonists are held in a lengthened position. And as you learned in Section One of this book, holding muscles in a stretched position for as little as thirty seconds actually inhibits them. So, with that in mind, ponder this one question. What do you think happens when you hold muscles in a stretched position 24/7? You could ask the infraspinatus and the teres minor. But if you have an Upper Cross Syndrome like most triathletes, these tiny rotator-cuff muscles responsible for lateral rotation of the shoulder have probably already given you a painful answer.

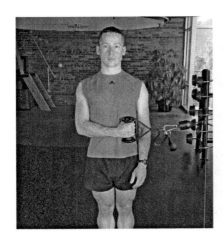

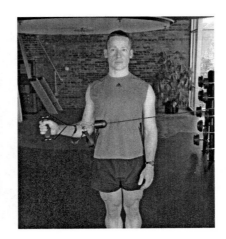

You need to give these lateral shoulder rotators some attention and strengthen them appropriately if they're to handle the demands of triathlon. All of the dynamic stabilizers can easily become fatigued under the swimming loads of the typical triathlete. In absence of proper conditioning, stability requirements get shifted to the static structures of the shoulder joint (i.e., the ligaments and cartilage of the joint capsule) as the dynamic stabilizers cross their threshold for strength and endurance. This leads to excessive wear and trauma to these inherently slow-healing tissues. External shoulder rotation exercises, like the one shown on the previous page, will target the key lateral rotators: the infraspinatus and the teres minor.

Yet tempo will be critical in the proper execution of the movement. The rotator cuff works *eccentrically* to stabilize the head of the humerus in the glenoid cavity. In laymen's terms, this means these muscles keep your arm from flying out of the socket every time you throw it above your head and grab a handful of water when you swim. Thus, the SAID principle discussed earlier in Section Two would demand that particular attention be paid to the eccentric or negative portion of any movement targeting the rotator cuff. Most studies would concur. Since maximum stress is placed on the muscle-tendon unit during eccentric loading, exercises which prove most beneficial for building the necessary resiliency to withstand such movements must emphasize the negative. Additionally, the majority of research demonstrates that eccentric strength transfers well to concentric strength, but the reverse is not typically true. So I recommend a 1-0-10 tempo where 1 equals one second for the concentric movement, 0 means there's no pause at end range of motion, and 10 equals ten seconds for the negative as you return your arm to the starting position. A weight which allows a minimum of twenty reps will seem easy at first. But by the end of the set, the endurance of the lateral rotators will be sufficiently tested.

149

Muscular imbalance in the shoulder rotators are often coupled with coordination deficits in the dynamic stabilizers, too. As muscles get pulled out of their ideal length-tension relationships, their timing can be adversely affected so that they try to work when they shouldn't. Instead of working in concert together, individual muscles fire before they should, while others fire a bit too late. The effect of this uncoordinated movement pattern is similar to what would happen if I tried to fill in for the conductor of the New York Symphony. I'd point to the clarinets when the trombones were supposed to play, and the whole orchestra would sound worse than a middle-school marching band. In your shoulder, this scenario plays out with impingement syndromes and other symptoms of instability characteristic of static and dynamic stabilizers which have not learned to perform the movement (i.e., the music) properly.

The Body Blade is an excellent tool to teach the shoulder stabilizers to work in concert with each other. Designed to oscillate up to 270 times a minute, it uses inertia to work the muscles in a sequenced fashion. Fatigue, often due to inexperience or lack of local muscular endurance and coordination, makes moving the Body Blade rhythmically virtually impossible. But consistent practice with this ingenious piece of equipment helps the dynamic stabilizers of the shoulder to develop the strength *and timing* needed for a lifetime of healthy strokes in the pool.

Example Movements:

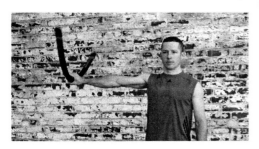

Hold the Bodyblade along the x-axis with one hand positioned to your side at shoulder level, palm down. Oscillate superior/inferior.

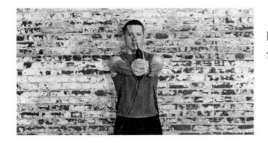

Hold the Bodyblade along the y-axis with two hands positioned in front of you at shoulder level, palms in. Oscillate medial/lateral.

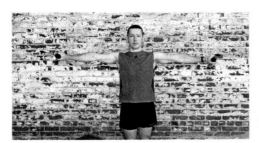 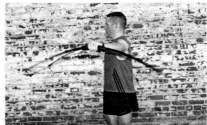 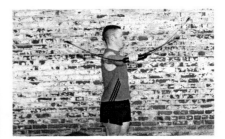

Hold two Bodyblades in each hand along the x-axis with arms positioned to your sides at shoulder level, palms down. Oscillate superior/inferior as you alternately rotate your torso to the right and to the left.

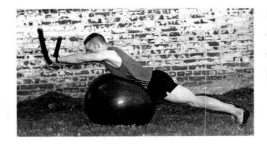

Lying across a physio ball in the prone position, hold the Bodyblade along the x-axis with both arms positioned above your head, palms down. Oscillate superior/inferior while maintaining your balance/ position on the ball.

Lying across a physio ball in the prone position, hold the Bodyblade along the x-axis with arm positioned 45 degrees to the body, palm down. Oscillate superior/inferior while maintaining your balance/position on the ball.

An alternative exercise I often use for clients who don't have a Body Blade is performed with a ball of minimal weight. Positioned next to a wall as shown in the figure below, the client internally rotates the arm to throw the ball against the wall. As the ball rebounds off the wall, the client catches it, externally rotating the arm. This movement is performed as smoothly as possible for time, building up to three minutes with the affected side. And though the number of repetitions will likely not be as high as with the Body Blade, the volume of work as the client progresses is sufficient to accomplish the same goal of healthy and well-timed shoulder musculature.

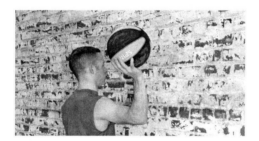 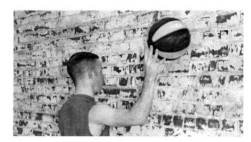

Cycling and the Back

We spend so much of our lives in flexion. We sit for work. We sit to relax. We sit to eat or drive. We even sleep in the fetal position at times. And cyclists take all this flexion up a notch. In order to get as aero as possible, the rider assumes a flexed posture. Then, this same cyclist will spend countless hours *strengthening* himself in the flexed position, thus ingraining this posture into his neuromuscular system. Soon the body doesn't know what extension is. I've assessed clients, many of them competitive cyclists or triathletes, whose thoracic curvatures were so excessive or whose lumbar curvatures were so lacking that it seemed they had forgotten how to extend the spine. That's a problem.

And if addressed early enough, the solution is simple. Body work in the form of mobilizations and myofascial release along with addressing workplace and home ergonomics go a long way toward restoring the ability to extend the spine. The myofascial work can be accomplished with a skilled massage therapist or A.R.T. practitioner. But I recommend a 4" foam roller for the thoracic and lumbar mobilizations as described below.

Foam Roller Horizontal Thoracic Mobilization

1. Lie on your side with a foam roller at armpit level perpendicular to your body.

2. Roll onto the foam roller so that you are supine (face up) with your glutes and feet on the floor. Fingers should be interlaced with your hands behind your head for support. Tongue should be on the roof of the mouth behind the teeth. The foam roller should be positioned across your thoracic spine.

3. Inhale as you extend over the foam roller and hold that position for 3-5 seconds.

4. Exhale and lower your shoulders to the floor.

5. Inhale as you return to the neutral position and repeat up to 3 times.

6. Move up (or down) to the next vertebra (while maintaining a neutral spine) and repeat the process. Focus on your specific areas of restriction.

7. When finished, roll off the foam roller onto your side, reversing the movement you made to get onto the roller.

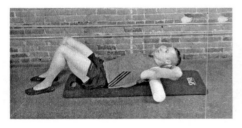 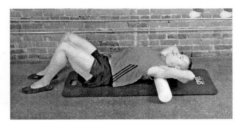

An active version of the above exercise called the **Seated Thoracic Mobilization** can be performed like so:

1. Sit on a physio ball or a low bench facing a wall with tongue on the roof of the mouth behind the teeth. Toes and knees should be on the wall.

2. Interlace your fingers and place your forearms and palms on the wall, resting your forehead on the backs of fingers. An alternative (and more aggressive) position places your elbows on the wall and the hands, palms facing, behind the head. Pushing the hands apart with the fingertips increases the external rotation.

3. Using the wall to assist you, actively extend the thoracic spine by pushing your chest toward the wall while pulling the elbows up and back.

4. Inhale as you extend, making sure to keep the chin tucked so as not to extend the cervical spine.

5. Hold the extension for 5-10 seconds and release.

6. Repeat for 5-10 reps, trying to go a bit deeper into extension every time.

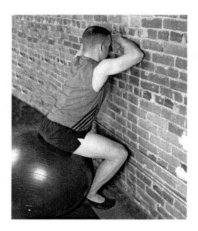 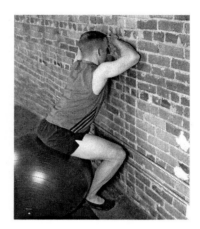

An excellent mobilization for the lumbar spine can be performed in a fashion similar to the thoracic mobilization above.

Foam Roller Horizontal Lumbar Mobilization

1. Lie on your side with a foam roller at navel level perpendicular to your body.

2. Roll onto the foam roller so that you are supine (face up) with your glutes and feet on the floor. Fingers should be interlaced with your hands behind your head for support. Tongue should be on the roof of the mouth behind the teeth. The foam roller should be positioned across your lumbar spine.

153

3. Inhale as you extend over the foam roller and hold that position for 3-5 seconds.

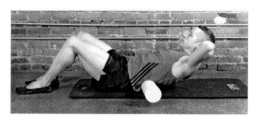

4. Exhale and lower your shoulders to the floor.

5. Inhale as you return to the neutral position and repeat up to 3 times.

6. Move up (or down) to the next vertebra (while maintaining a neutral spine) and repeat the process. Focus on your specific areas of restriction.

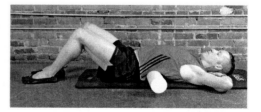

7. When finished, roll off the foam roller onto your side, reversing the movement you made to get onto the roller.

Note: People with a diagnosis of ankylosing spondylitis should not perform any of the above mobilizations. Also, if you have a history of dizziness when your neck is in extension, you should be cleared by a physician before performing the foam-roller mobilizations as this could be a sign of vertebral artery occlusion.

A final movement which is simple to perform yet very effective at mobilizing the spine is one I recommend after prolonged sitting in a chair, a long bike ride, or any extended period of flexion. It is called the **McKenzie press-Up**.

1. Lie in a **prone** position (face down) with your hands positioned outside your shoulders, palm down.

2. Exhale and push your chest off the floor. Make sure to keep your ASIS (hip bones) in contact with the floor at all times, even if this means your arms do not fully extend. Keep your glutes and back muscles relaxed. I like to take a big diaphragmatic breath in to help stretch the rectus abdominus. Sometimes I'll twist left to focus on the right side or twist right to focus on the left side.

3. Return to start position and repeat for five to ten repetitions.

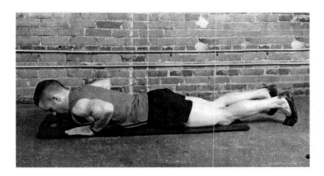 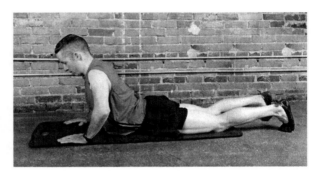

As mentioned earlier, proper abdominal development and function is essential to the integrity of the spine. So, in addition to consistent myofascial work, mobilizations, and increased postural awareness, the Prehab and Postural Correction phase of weights includes a renewed emphasis on core conditioning. After all, the legs and arms are obviously not being neglected with swimming, cycling, and running. Yet a triathlete's static stabilizers, which have growing demands placed upon them as the season progresses, often get sacrificed in a training program as the volume of the other three disciplines increases. This is a critical mistake as static stability is the foundation for dynamic stability.

So, much of the work now will focus on static stability: The ability to hold the body in any position that allows one to carry out a given task (i.e., a triathlon) against the load of the extremities or any other force. You'll still follow the concept of lowers before obliques before uppers in regard to strengthening the abdominals. But now the exercises will be completed with time as a goal rather than repetitions, in an effort to improve postural endurance. Failure to adequately develop this ability will result in premature fatigue in the muscular system, ultimately resulting in pathological loading of the ligamentous system, pain, and cessation of training.

A movement which is purposefully included in this phase is an exercise called **Horse-Stance Vertical**. I'll admit it's tedious. But it's very effective at overriding any neurological inhibition the body may have due to pain or sensory motor amnesia. It's one of the movements I used to rehab myself from the back injury I wrote about in Section Two. It targets the multifidus, a muscle of the back and a key player in segmental stability of the spine. And though most of you, if asked, couldn't consciously activate your multifidi if a Kona slot depended on it, this exercise can help you turn on that muscle and get it working to protect your back again.

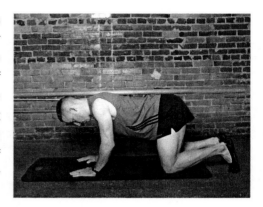

1. Get on your hands and knees with your hands directly beneath your shoulders and your knees directly beneath your hips. Bend your arms slightly at the elbow so that your back is parallel to the floor. I recommend you use a dowel to ensure you maintain a neutral spine. The dowel rod should touch your sacrum, your thoracic spine between your shoulder blades, and the back of your head as shown in the figure above.

2. Draw your TVA in toward your spine and activate your pelvic floor musculature. (Women: Perform a kegel. Men: Pull your testicles up toward your head.)

3. Lift one hand and the contralateral knee off the floor just enough to slip a piece of paper under it. If I were looking at you from the side, I should hardly be able to tell you're moving at all.

4. Remain still, deviating neither side to side nor fore and aft, and hold this position for 5-10 seconds.

5. Repeat this procedure on the opposite sides, again holding for 5-10 seconds. Continue alternating sides for 8-10 reps each side.

155

Simply put, this exercise puts a diagonal shear force through the spine which the body senses as dangerous (and, indeed, under most conditions it is). Thus, the neuromuscular system activates any previously dormant muscles which are necessary to maintain the orthopedic integrity essential to perform the movement safely. I will often program one shorter set of this movement into my client's strength-training routine prior to lifts such as squats or dead lifts to make sure the multifidi are turned on and ready to assist with stabilizing the back.

Two final exercises which are highly effective, both for building sport-specific positional endurance as well as countering the postural aberrations inherent to triathlon, are the **bent-over row** and the **prone cobra**. Both movements work on postural endurance and are excellent choices in a triathlete's program to alleviate some of the muscular imbalances typical of the sport. But the bent-over row is one with a high degree of transfer to the bike, as illustrated in the photographs below.

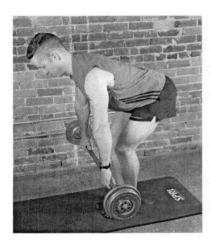 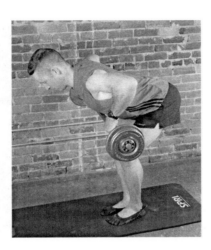

BENT-OVER ROW

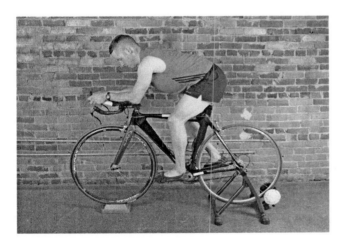

CYCLIST ON BIKE

1. Stand with feet pedal-width apart holding a pair of dumbbells or a bar with a pronated grip, chest out, shoulders back, navel in.

2. Soften your knees (approximately 20° bend), which makes the iliotibial band taut so that the gluteus maximus has a foundation off which to work. The glutes can then help share the load so that the back need not work in isolation.

3. Pivot forward at the hips so that the torso is positioned between 45 and 90° in relation to the legs. The angle should be dictated by the flexibility in the hamstrings—if your back starts to round or you lose your neutral lumbar and thoracic curves, you have bent over too much. Head should remain in neutral, too, (i.e., don't look forward), to avoid shortening the sub occipitals.

4. Pull weight to chest while maintaining high elbows, pausing at the top of the movement. The forearms and wrist should remain perpendicular to the floor.

5. Return the weight to start position and repeat for the designated number of reps.

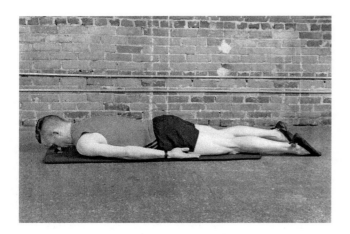 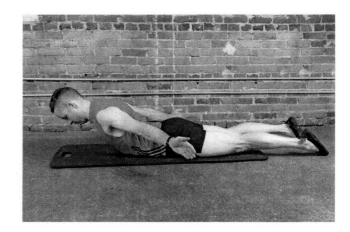

PRONE COBRA

1. Lie in the prone position (navel down) with arms by your side, palms up.

2. Inhale and lift the chest off the ground, aiming to reverse your thoracic curvature as you supinate your arms and squeeze your shoulder blades together. Keep the lower body relaxed with feet on the floor. *Those whose lumbar curvature is excessive should concentrate on initiating the movement by squeezing the glutes first so that recruitment of the lumbar erectors is not excessive.* Make sure chin stays tucked so that head is aligned with the rest of the spine to avoid shortening of the sub occipitals.

3. Hold for the designated period of time.

Running and the Ankle, the Knee, and the Hip

Running is essentially eccentric. And I don't mean that runners are odd (they have nothing on triathletes). What I mean is that the impact of running is handled by the body eccentrically. The muscles contract and lengthen at the same time as they control the weight of the body in its descent back to earth. See, what comes up eventually comes down—at two to seven times body weight depending on the speed and form of the runner. And this load must be eccentrically controlled ninety times per minute per leg! Thus, just like the rotator cuff must be conditioned appropriately to handle the demands of swimming, training for the lower-body triple extensors must include an emphasis on the negative portion of a lift so nothing in the kinetic chain eventually fails.

Calf-Raise Negatives

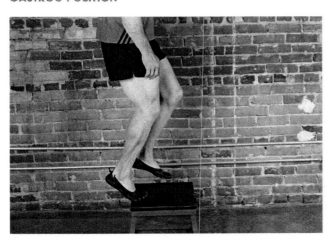
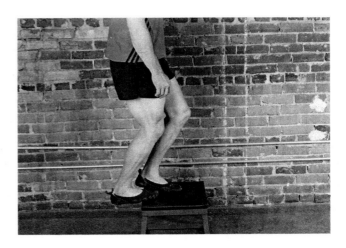

GASTROC POSITION

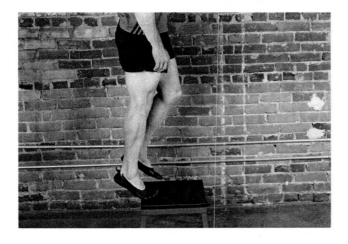
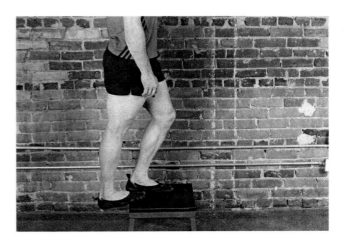

SOLEUS POSITION

1. Stand with the balls of your feet on a step and your heels hanging off.

2. Rise up onto toes using both legs.

3. Take the dominant leg away and use a 10-count to control your descent so that your heel ends up below the ball of your foot.

4. At end range of motion, put your dominant leg back on the step and rise back up to the top position again, repeating the process for the designated number of reps.

5. Doing the movement with a straight leg targets the gastrocnemius. Doing the movement with a bent knee (15-20°) targets the soleus. Both versions should be performed.

The next two exercises are excellent ones to include in the triathlete's program as they work unilaterally in all three planes of motion to strengthen muscles which become weak in relation to their antagonists. Performing them correctly will result in not only a stronger leg, but a smarter leg. And a smart leg is a fast leg—exactly what you want for the final miles of a triathlon.

159

Unilateral Supine Hip-Extension

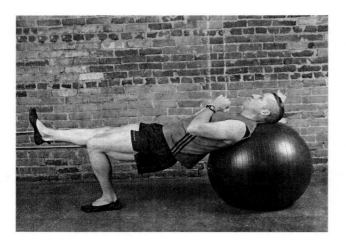 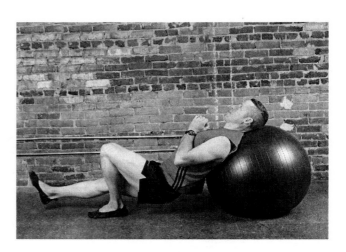

1. Seated on a physio ball, roll yourself down until the ball supports your head and shoulders. You should have your feet on the ground with your shins perpendicular to the floor. Your arms can be out at your side like a tightrope walker or, as proficiency allows, closer to your body until they are crossed over your chest. Maintain TVA function (i.e., navel drawn in slightly) to avoid over-recruitment of the lumbar erectors.

2. Take the dominant leg away from the floor by extending your knee to keep the leg parallel with the ground.

3. Lower your glutes toward the floor while maintaining a perpendicular shin of the leg on the ground.

4. Push through your heel as you raise your pelvis back to the start position, making sure to contract the glute in addition to the hamstring and the lower back. The last inch of the movement in the elevated position may be the most difficult, but it is equally important.

5. Repeat for the designated number of reps before repeating on the opposite side.

NOTE: If one glute seems not to be firing as well as the other, gently tap or touch the glute to increase your sensory awareness of the muscle. If you are still having difficulty getting the glute to fire, stretch the psoas on that side as it may be tonic and stealing some of the neural drive meant for that muscle.

Unilateral Supine Hip-Extension Knee Flexion

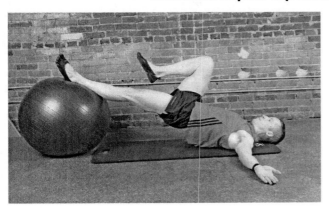 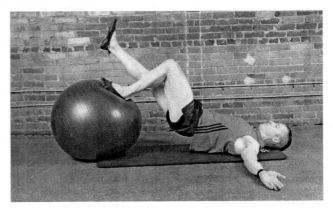

UNILATERAL SUPINE HIP-EXTENSION KNEE FLEXION

1. Lie supine and place your legs on a physio ball with your arms out at your side palms up, perpendicular to the body. Activate your TVA (draw your navel in slightly) to avoid over-recruitment of the lumbar erectors.

2. Lift your pelvis off the ground by contracting your glutes in addition to your lower back and hamstrings, until your shoulders, hip, and ankles are in line.

3. Take the dominant leg away while keeping your pelvis level and in an elevated position.

4. Flex your knee and pull your heel toward your glute as far as you can.

5. Extend the leg to return the ball to the start position.

6. Repeat for the designated number of reps before repeating on the opposite side.

NOTE: Putting less leg on the ball (i.e., your heels instead of your calves) as well as bringing your arms closer toward your body to decrease your base of support will make the exercise more challenging. Also, both the Unilateral Supine Hip-Extension and the Unilateral Supine Hip-Extension Knee Flexion can be performed with two legs if skill level and strength necessitate additional support or balance. Transitioning between two-legged support and one-legged support can be accomplished with the aid of a dowel rod as shown in the pictures below.

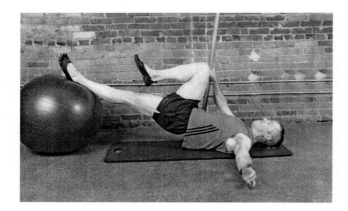 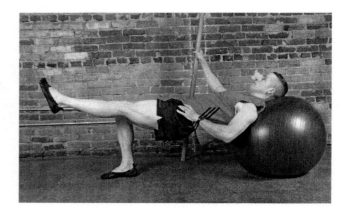

WITH SUPPORT

This last exercise works many different muscles, but the focus is on strengthening the glute medius. The glute medius is a frontal plane stabilizer of critical importance to gait. To prove this to yourself, try the following experiment:

Take a normal step and note how long the step is.

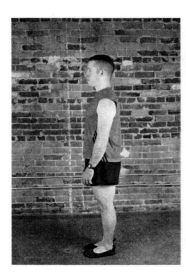 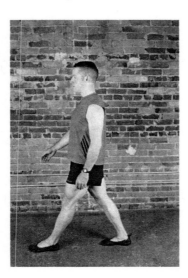

Now push your hip to the side of the leg you stepped with previously, and take another step.

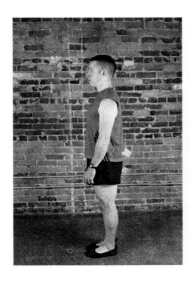 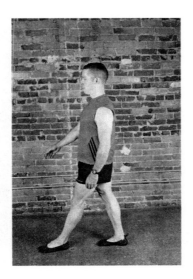

Your stride length was noticeably shorter. Since run speed is determined by both stride rate and stride length, you can see how running with what is essentially a Trendelenburg sign is going to make you slower. Additionally, the quadratus lumborum (QL) must now work to hike the hip on the other side to allow enough room for the leg to come through during the swing phase of gait. This often results in back pain as the QL gets overworked, not to mention all of the orthopedic wear and tear as a consequence of faulty alignment. The exercise below effectively targets the commonly neglected glute medius. And, again, it strengthens it both concentrically and eccentrically.

Oblique Raise Abductor Negatives

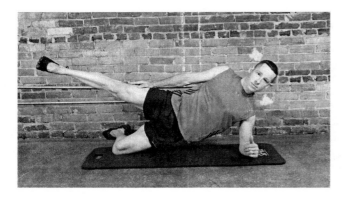 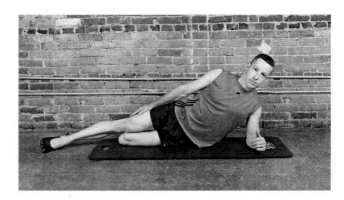

1. Lie on your side with your underneath leg bent 90° at the knee and your underneath arm directly under your shoulder and bent at the elbow, so that your forearm extends in out in front of you perpendicular to your body.

2. Lift your pelvis off the ground while at the same time abducting your leg into the air as far as possible while still maintaining perfect alignment of the underneath knee, hip, and shoulder. Do not allow the elevated leg to either bend at the knee or flex forward at the hip.

3. Descend back to the start position using a slow, controlled tempo of approximately six to ten seconds.

4. Repeat for the designated number of reps before repeating on the opposite side.

163

Prehab and Postural Correction Phase Details

• % of 1 RM dependent on the exercise being performed

• 2-3 sets (2 sets closer to competition and NO LEGS 10-14 days prior to GOAL EVENT and NO ARMS 7-10 days prior to GOAL EVENT)

• 30-60 seconds between sets

• Repetition scheme dependent on the exercise being performed

• Once every fourteen days, alternating with SM phase (i.e., one week of PPC followed by one week of SM)

• Perform the exercises with the highest degree of neurological complexity or axial loading first

• 60 minutes approximate workout time

1. Exercise targeting your current/historic injury site or weak/problem area (i.e., swim and shoulder, bike and back, or run and ankle, knee, or hip). If you have more than one, perform the one with the highest degree of neurological complexity or axial loading first. Thus, you may choose three different areas here for the run, plus exercises for both swim and bike for a total of nine exercises during this workout. If your orthopedic history is clean, focus on the discipline which is currently your weakest. Superset with exercise #2 below.

2. Lower Abdominal superset with exercise #1 above.

3. Oblique Abdominal.

4. Upper Abdominal superset with exercise #5 below.

5. Back-Extension (found in the BEND PATTERN section) superset with exercise #4 above.

Exercises	Sets	Rest	Reps	Intensity	Tempo/ Duration
Bent-Over Row Maintain lordosis and HIGH elbows. Superset with Unilateral Calf Raise below.	2-3	n/a	20-30	1 RR	1-3-1
Unilateral Calf Raise with Negatives Alternate between straight leg and bent leg.	2-3	60 sec	12-15 each	1 RR	Controlled negative
Unilateral Body Blade on One Leg Begin with Non-dominant side and switch legs each set.	2-3	n/a	20-30 sec each side	1 RR	Rhythmic
Lower Abdominal #2A Use a BP cuff for biofeedback.	2-3	60 sec	10-12 each side, alternating	1 RR or 40mmHg + 30mmHg	Slow/ controlled
Side Bridge with Ext Shoulder Rotation Keep shoulder glued to side.	2-3	45 sec	15-30 each	1 RR	Controlled negative
Stabilizer Ensure neutral spinal curvatures. Superset with Prone Cobra below.	2-3	n/a	1	1 RR	60-180s HOLD
Prone Cobra Keep chin tucked (don't look forward).	2-3	30 sec	1	1 RR	60-180s HOLD

CHAPTER 6:
The Exercises

NOTE: Each group of exercises is roughly listed in order of neurological demand from easiest to hardest. **Descents** (steps down in complexity so that the exercise can be performed in spite of injury and/or motor learning deficits) can be made if the primal pattern is deficient. However, they should only be used if necessary as a step toward mastering the baseline movement.

Additionally, all of the exercises can be performed statically, if pain precludes movement. The protocol then would be to find a position that does not elicit any discomfort, and hold it for a designated period of time (e.g., sixty seconds). Due to the body's unique ability to strengthen not only in the position held, but also 15°above and below the held position, pain-free range of motion should gradually increase. The athlete can then train in this new pain-free range of motion which will eventually increase in approximately 30° intervals until full movement is obtained. The critical concept to understand here is that if you are experiencing pain other than muscular discomfort, **something is wrong**—form, core function, flexibility, etc.—and needs to be addressed. A CHEK practitioner or someone skilled in corrective exercise should be able to determine the etiology of the problem.

One last item to note is that the below lists of exercises is not meant to be exhaustive—there are countless other movements which could benefit the triathlete and have not been included either for the sake of space or simplicity. Indeed, many of the exercises listed can be ascended, descended, or combined with others to create different ones with a different developmental focus. The key, then, is to always have a reason for performing a particular movement. If you cannot answer the question of why a specific exercise is in your program, then the answer is to question the inclusion of that exercise!

SQUAT

You don't know squat. But you should. One of the seven primal patterns, squatting was essential for survival when we were cavemen and -women. And while evolution has developed our Texting pattern such that many of us have a thenar eminence the size of our bicep, our squatting skills have suffered in kind. Because of this, over 80% of people will endure an episode of back pain in his or her lifetime. And triathletes aren't immune. So squat! It's good for your back. It's good for your knees. And it's good for your triathlon performance. The only thing it's not good for is your orthopedic surgeon's bank account.

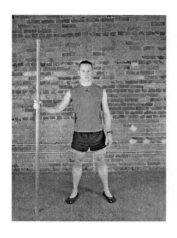
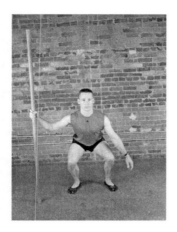

FIRST DESCENT—1 DOWEL-ROD SUPPORT

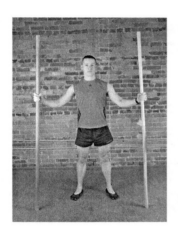
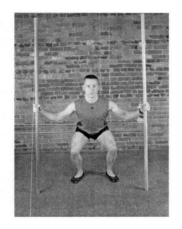

SECOND DESCENT—2 DOWEL-ROD SUPPORTS

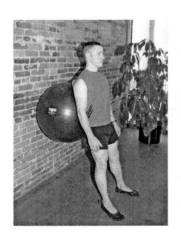
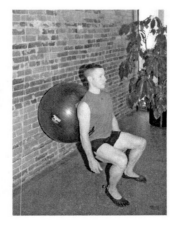

THIRD DESCENT—SWISS BALL ON WALL AS SUPPORT

EXAMPLE EXERCISES

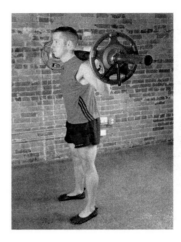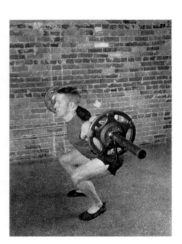

Benefits: Trains a movement pattern encountered in sport and essential for daily function. Strengthens almost every muscle in the body by integrating glutes, quadriceps, and hamstrings with core musculature.

Key Points: Chest out, shoulders back, navel in, eyes on horizon. Knees track over second toes of feet. Release air through pursed lips during the ascent.

BACK SQUAT

169

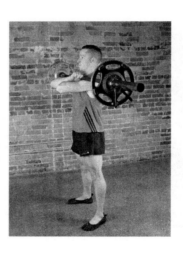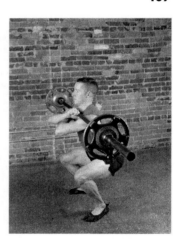

Benefits: Like back squat above. Also trains thoracic extension and allows for a more upright posture such that improper form is less likely.

Key Points: Same as back squat above.

FRONT SQUAT

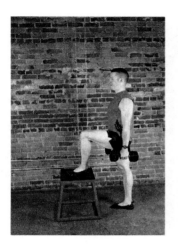 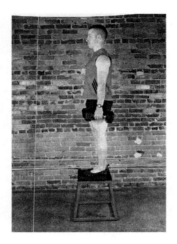

STEP UP

Benefits: Strengthens functional movement pattern closely resembling unilateral demands of BIKE/RUN with more emphasis on frontal and transverse plane musculature than exercises performed on two legs.

Key Points: Maintain perfect posture with TVA activation. Knee tracks over second toe. Keep pelvis level. Do not allow lateral hip deviation of stance leg. Push through heel.

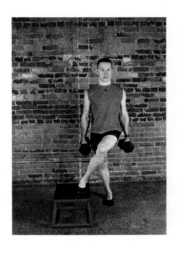 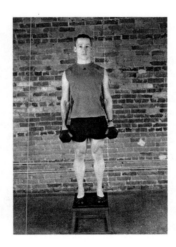 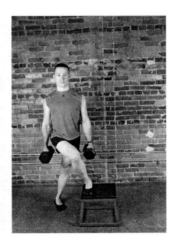

CROSSOVER STEP UP

Benefits: Same as Step Up above but with increased development and flexibility of the medial and lateral rotators of the hip.

Key Points: Maintain perfect posture with TVA activation. Knee tracks over second toe. Keep pelvis level. Do not allow lateral hip deviation of stance leg. Push through heel.

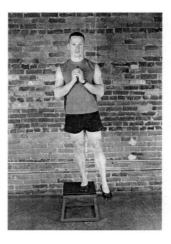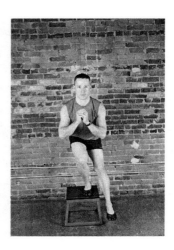

Benefits: Strengthen same muscles as squats above with greater requirement for frontal and transverse plane stability. Unilateral position more closely resembles demands of BIKE/RUN.

UNILATERAL SQUAT

Key Points: Maintain lordosis throughout movement as knee tracks over second toe. Push through heel.

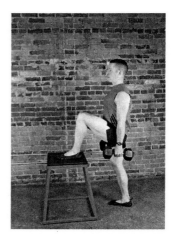

Benefits: Same as Step Up above with emphasis on glutes as quadriceps are put at a mechanical disadvantage. Higher requirement for knee and pelvic stability. Excellent choice for optimizing hill-specific RUN strength.

HIGH STEP UP

Key Points: Same as Step Up above with emphasis on pushing bench away from you rather than stepping onto the bench.

LUNGE

85% of gait takes place on one leg. Whether you're pedaling perfect circles or in squares like most novices, you're deriving most of your power from alternating legs while on the bike. Even swimming works the legs unilaterally. So while the squat pattern is a foundation for many movements in triathlon, the literal next step is the lunge. Performed correctly, it strengthens the hamstrings and the glutes—muscles often underdeveloped and underutilized on triathletes—as well as the quads. Additional benefits, from improved balance to ramped-up core recruitment, make this movement a critical one to master for the competitive triathlete.

NOTE: All of the lunge movements described below can be made more neurologically challenging and sport specific by adding arm movements such as bicep curls or shoulder presses. When doing so, always follow a **cross-crawl pattern** where the arm and the opposite leg work together. This will stimulate biomotor integration as well as help establish more connections in the corpus callosum, the part of the brain which connects the right hemisphere to the left hemisphere. Additionally, the Twist pattern can (and should when proficiency allows) be integrated into any of the lunge patterns below so that the legs learn to work in a coordinated fashion with the spine—as they should in the sport of triathlon and the sport of life!

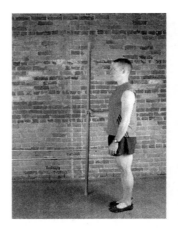
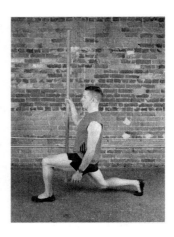

FIRST DESCENT—1 DOWEL-ROD SUPPORT

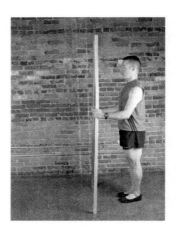
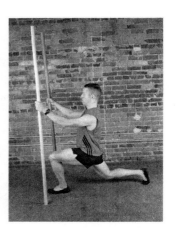

SECOND DESCENT—2 DOWEL-ROD SUPPORTS

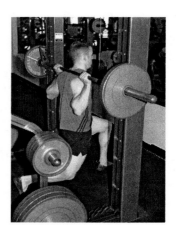

THIRD DESCENT—SMITH MACHINE

EXAMPLE EXERCISES

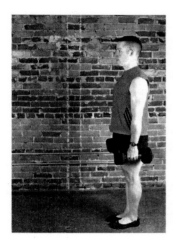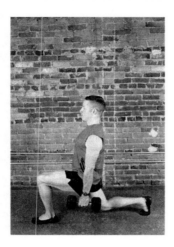

LUNGE

Benefits: Trains a movement pattern encountered in sports which closely resembles demands of BIKE/RUN with requirement to stabilize in three dimensions.

Key Points: Keep an upright posture with head up during bottom lunge position. Maintain pelvis in frontal plane. Shin of forward leg should be perpendicular to floor when thigh is parallel to floor. Knee of rear leg should **not** touch the ground. Focus on pushing through heel of forward leg rather than forefoot.

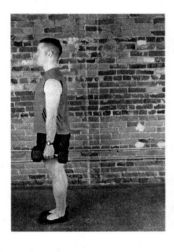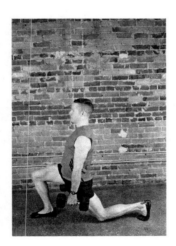

BACKWARD LUNGE

Benefits: Same as Lunge above with more core requirement because of altered vision as well as heightened proprioception and excitation of nervous system.

Key Points: Same as Lunge above with emphasis on maintaining an upright posture.

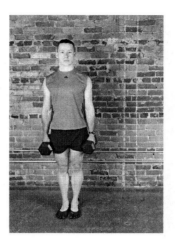
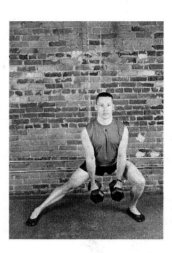

SIDE LUNGE

Benefits: Same as Lunge above with an emphasis on strengthening muscles working in the frontal plane.

Key Points: Maintain upright posture throughout movement as well as keeping feet and torso relatively square. The foot that you step away from does not roll but remains flat. The leg that you step away from is straight but **not** locked. If using a bar/dowel rod on the shoulders, keep it parallel with floor at all times.

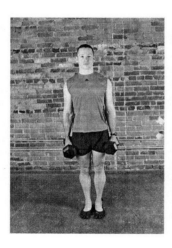
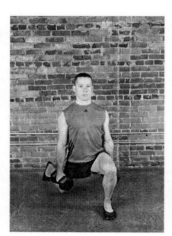
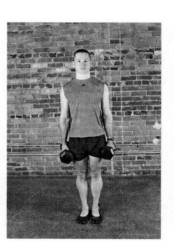
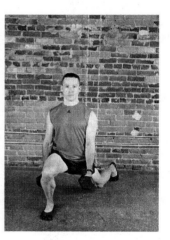

45° LUNGE

Benefits: Same as Side Lunge above.

Key Points: Keep forward foot and torso relatively square. Allow trailing leg to pivot off the ball of the foot to maintain integrity of knee as a hinge joint. Keep bar/dowel rod parallel with floor at all times if using one on the shoulders.

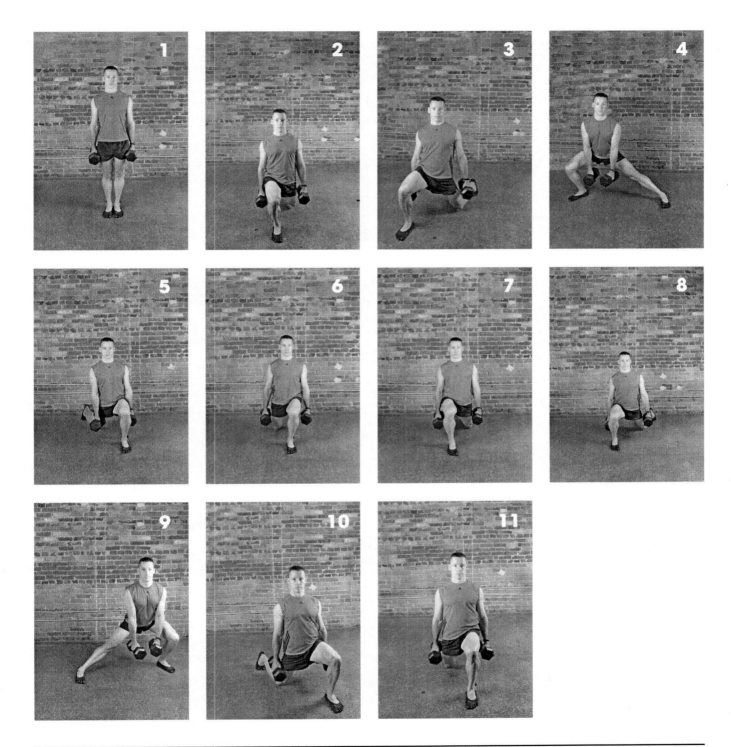

CLOCK LUNGE

Benefits: Same as all lunge forms above with work in all three planes of motion.

Key Points: Same as all Lunges above.

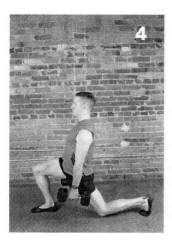 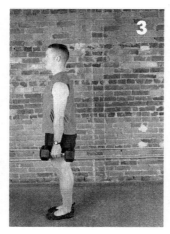 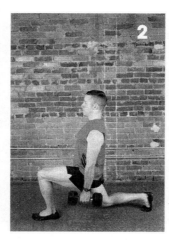 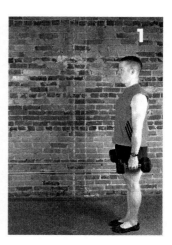

Benefits: Heightens neural excitation as lunge musculature is strengthened in a mobile three-dimensional environment which more closely resembles the demands of RUNNING.

Key Points: Same as Lunge above but moving.

LUNGE WALK

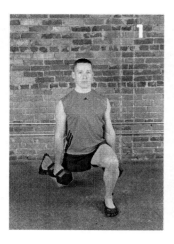 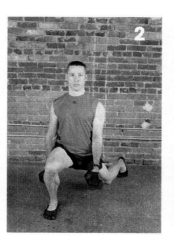 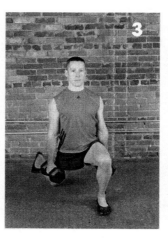 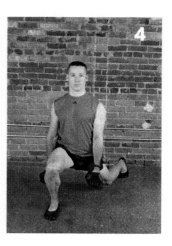

Benefits: Same as Lunge Walk above with increased complexity, neural excitation, and force production as well as stabilization in the frontal plane.

Key Points: Same as 45° Lunge above.

45° LUNGE WALK

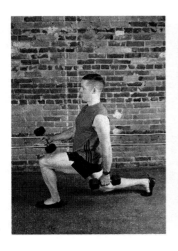
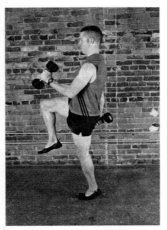

RUN POSE

Benefits: Strengthens RUN-specific musculature while addressing both dynamic and static stability.

Key Points: Hold top position before returning to the start position. Do not allow torso to collapse forward when in lunge position.

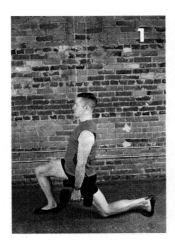
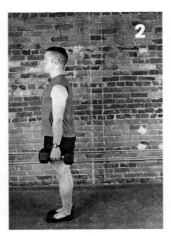
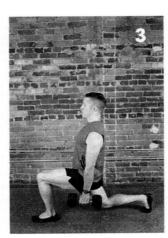
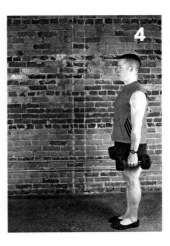

BACKWARD LUNGE WALK

Benefits: Heightens neural excitation and core requirement/proprioception due to altered vision status as lunge musculature is strengthened in a mobile, three-dimensional environment which more closely resembles the demands of RUNNING.

Key Points: Same as Lunge Walk above with emphasis on maintenance of an upright posture.

Why lunge or do any movement backwards? Well, you never know when proficiency in a seemingly unnecessary movement will help you make the finish line. My 2007 return to IMLP almost ended badly. But as the following excerpt from my race report shows, thorough preparation which leaves no training stone unturned is the hallmark of a successful triathlete:

A sharp pain and the forest of signs faded as all my attention went to my left leg threatening to cramp. That damn gracillis again—the only way to stretch it was to go into a side lunge to the right. As soon as I did that, my right psoas and quad turned into concrete and then the chain reaction began. I stood back up, but the gracillis locked down again as random contractions forced me to stop in an awkward position. A couple of volunteers saw me struggling in the middle of the road and came over to help me with words of motivation. A muscle relaxer is what I needed more as I eased into a side lunge once again. I wondered if the camera crew was getting this. Linda, one of the producers, has always wanted to capture this moment. "Drama," she calls it. Immobilization is what it felt like. I stood there petrified as the two men I ran down a couple of miles back passed me. I tried to move forward when my muscles finally relaxed, but they seized up again. "God," I prayed, "please just let me finish." The volunteer told me there was an aid station just up the road. As I looked ahead, all I could see was my competition fading further and further into the distance. I looked behind me and saw Jeff and the camera crew a couple of hundred yards away. They obviously didn't see me or they would have been circling like vultures. It's not that they wanted "drama." But if it happened while they were near, they had strict instructions from Linda to capture it on film.

Parts of my brain's neurons are filled with the origins, insertions, and actions of certain muscles. I used a few of those to convince me to try walking backwards. I felt stupid doing it, but I was making forward progress for the first time in several minutes. "I'll do this the whole way if necessary," I thought. "Hell, I can turn around at the last moment for the finish-line camera if I have to." So I moved forward... while backwards... and talked to the two volunteers as I walked at a twenty-minute/mile pace. When I tried to turn around, I was rewarded by no cramps. Eventually, I thanked the volunteers for their company and broke into a slow jog. Twinges brushed across my body like cobwebs, but left me alone if I ran more with my arms and let my legs just be along for the ride. Only when I changed my arm swing to grab nutrition at an aid station did my legs protest enough to alter my stride.

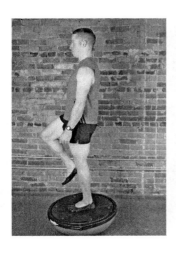 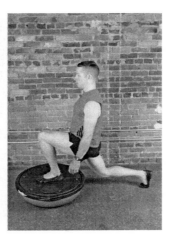

BOSU LUNGE

Benefits: Heightens neural excitation and core requirement/ proprioception due to unstable surface. Particularly applicable to off-road triathletes who must RUN on dirt or sand.

Key Points: Same as lunge above.

PULL

Another one of the seven primal patterns, pulling movements are often neglected or underdeveloped compared to their sister pattern, pushing movements. This is often because people don't have vision for what they can't see. When you "see" a tree, you don't really see the whole tree. You don't see its roots. You don't see the other side of the trunk or the top of the canopy. Yet the tree could never be fully developed without them. So just because you can't see the muscles of your posterior chain does not mean you should ignore them. You are more than just your mirror muscles. In fact, it is the predominance of anterior chain movements in triathlon which make pulling proficiency so important for triathletes to maintain postural balance along with orthopedic health.

NOTE: Anytime you do unilateral (i.e. single arm) Pull or Push Patterns, you are creating a rotational force and, thus, mobilizing the spine. This not only helps nourish the spine by pumping the spinal discs with the fluids essential for health, it's also specific to the movement patterns involved in triathlon.

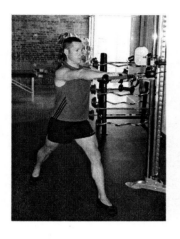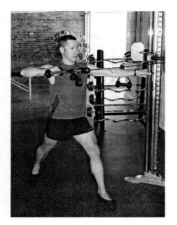

FIRST DESCENT—BRACED

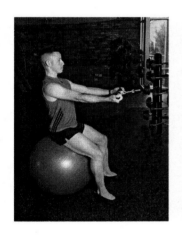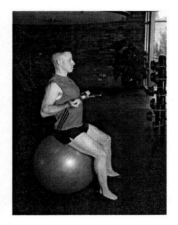

SECOND DESCENT—SEATED OR LYING

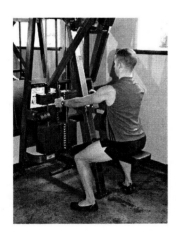

THIRD DESCENT—SEATED OR LYING ON FIXED-AXIS MACHINE

EXAMPLE EXERCISES

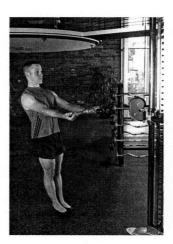 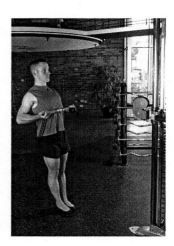

Benefits: Strengthens key musculature which aid in countering some of the postural deviations incurred through the sport of triathlon. Trains some of the prime movers in SWIMMING as well as the arm muscles which aid in climbing on the BIKE and proper hill RUNNING. Proper scapular adductor and scapular humeral muscles activation is trained also.

LOW ROW

Key Points: Maintain chest out, shoulders back, and navel in throughout movement. Scapula and arm movement should terminate at the same time.

183

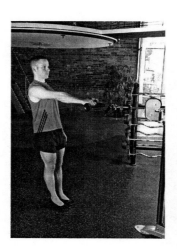 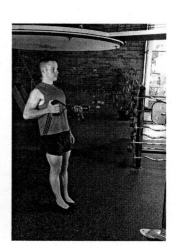

Benefits: Same as Low Row above in a unilateral environment which more closely resembles the demands and upper-body movement patterns in SWIMMING, CYCLING, and RUNNING with greater activation of musculature responsible for movement and stabilization in the transverse plane. Particularly beneficial in reversing excessive thoracic kyphosis.

UNILATERAL ROW

Key Points: Maintain palm in. Keep core square. Terminate scapula and arm movement at the same time.

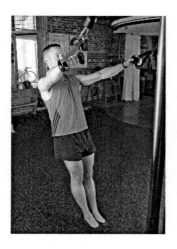 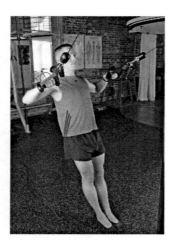

HIGH ROW

Benefits: Strengthens the external shoulder rotators with modest recruitment of the entire extensor chain. The standing position has a high degree of carryover to the RUN and is a good alternative for athletes unable to maintain a lordotic position during the bent-over row (see below in BEND section) due to inexperience or lack of body awareness.

Key Points: Maintain TVA activation and high elbows throughout movement. Do not allow wrists to flex and over- utilize the forearm flexors.

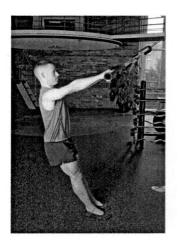 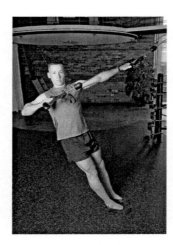 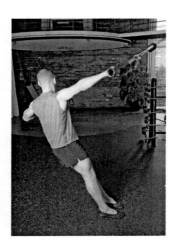

HIGH ROW
WITH ROTATION

Benefits: Same as High Row above coupled with Twist Pattern development as found in the SWIM.

Key Points: Same as High Row above. Initiate movement with twist rather than pull.

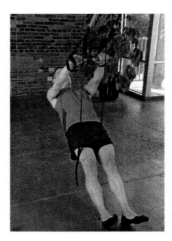 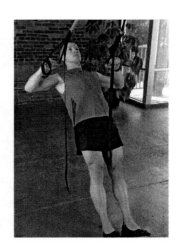

Benefits: Same as High Row above, but as a *closed-chain* exercise which better transfers to the SWIM.   **SUSPENDED ROW**
Good transitional exercise for those who lack the strength to perform Pull Ups or Chin Ups.

Key Points: Same as High Row above.

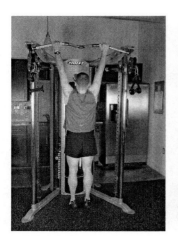 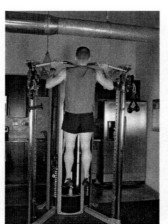 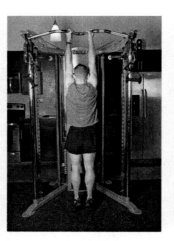 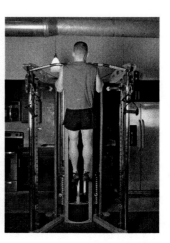

Benefits: Same as Low Row above with additional emphasis on latissimus dorsi development which is   **PULL UPS/CHIN UPS**
crucial in its role as a connection between the lumbar spine and the arms as well as its communication
with the contra-lateral glute. A *closed-chain* exercise which better transfers to SWIM-specific strength.

Key Points: For Pull Ups—maintain forearms perpendicular to floor at all times to avoid internal rotation
of the shoulders, which would perpetuate postural distortions incurred through the sport of triathlon.

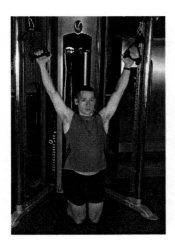 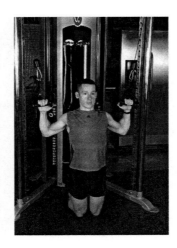

OVERHAND PULL DOWN   **Benefits:** Same as Pull Ups above but as an *open-chain* exercise.

Key Points: Same as Pull Ups above.

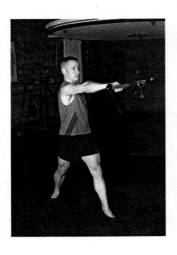 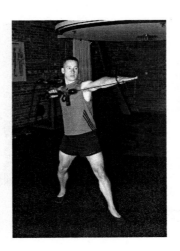

CABLE PULLS   **Benefits:** Trains TVA activation while improving core stabilization, with arm moments similar to those which occur during the SWIM, out-of-the-saddle CYCLING, and the RUN.

Key Points: Maintain good posture and TVA activation throughout. Scapula and arm motion should terminate at the same time.

Varied stances (ordered from least difficult to most difficult):

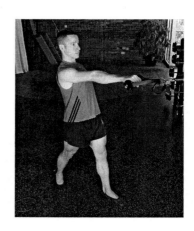

COUNTER STANCE

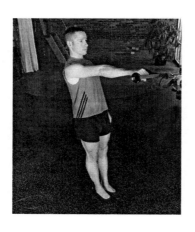

PARALLEL STANCE

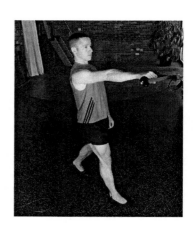

IPSILATERAL STANCE

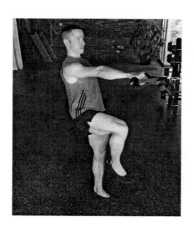

SINGLE LEG CONTRALATERAL

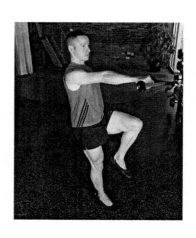

SINGLE LEG IPSILATERAL

PUSH

In reality, muscles do not push. Movements, even pushing ones, occur because a muscle (or muscles) contracts or shortens and *pulls* the origin and insertion together. Even during a push up, the triceps contract to *pull* the origin and insertion closer together, causing the arms to extend and the body to rise away from the ground. This, of course, is achieved with the help of additional actions of the pectorals and deltoids (not to mention countless core muscles essential to a proper push up. These are the same muscles often lacking in a guy who has a 250-pound bench, yet can't hold his pelvis level to perform a decent push up). In the sport of triathlon, forward propulsion is achieved mainly by the action of muscles which "push". This section will focus exclusively on the upper-body pushing movements.

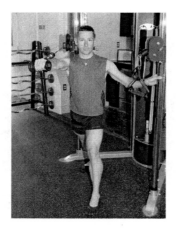

FIRST DESCENT—BRACED

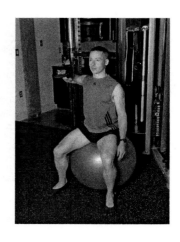

SECOND DESCENT—SEATED OR LYING

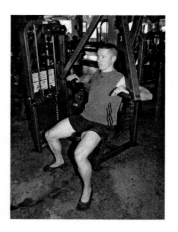

THIRD DESCENT—SEATED OR LYING ON FIXED-AXIS MACHINE

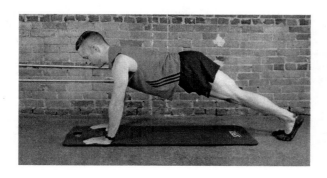

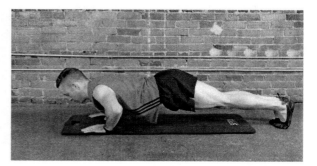

Benefits: Strengthens pectorals, anterior deltoids, and triceps while working key postural muscles which are activated in order to support the pelvis.

Key Points: Lead with the chest but do not let it touch floor, as this will overstress the anterior capsule of the shoulder joint. Maintain support of pelvis at all times and do not allow head to fall out of alignment with the spine.

PUSH UPS

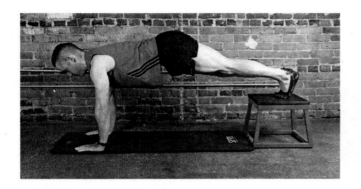 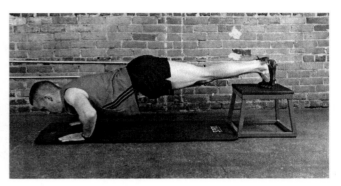

DECLINE PUSH UPS **Benefits:** Same as Push Ups above, with higher intensity due to the increased demand placed on all working musculature as the different angle results in a greater load put on the body.

Key Points: Same as Push Ups above with greater focus on **not** allowing the pelvis to drop.

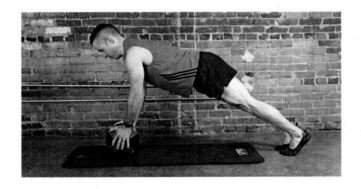 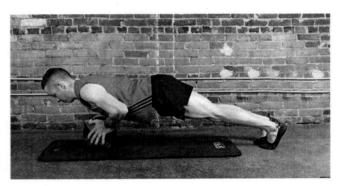

MEDICINE-BALL PUSH UPS **Benefits:** Same as Push Ups above with a higher emphasis on the triceps and greater demand placed on the shoulder stabilizers since the ball has the potential to move.

Key Points: Same as Push Ups above.

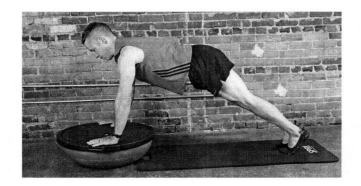
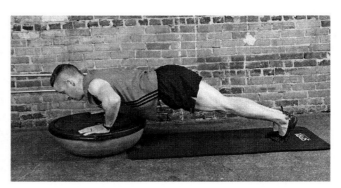

Benefits: Same as Push Ups above with greater stabilizer stimulus required when working in an unstable environment, which also demands more equal force production from both arms.

Key Points: Same as Push Ups above.

191

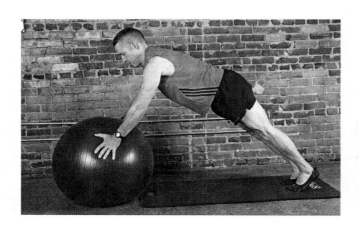
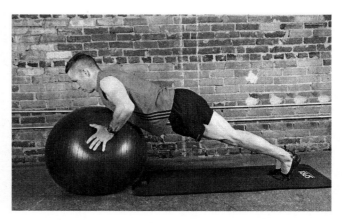

Benefits: Same as Bosu Push Ups above.

Key Points: Same as Push Ups above.

HANDS-ON-PHYSIO-BALL
PUSH UPS

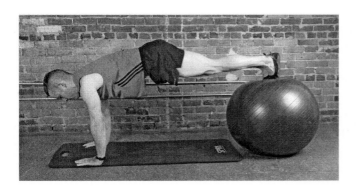 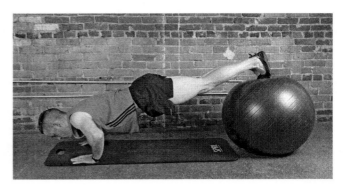

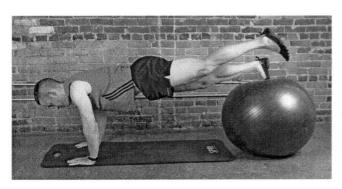 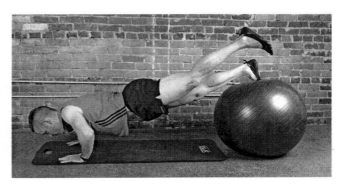

FEET-ON-PHYSIO-BALL PUSH UPS

Benefits: Same as Bosu Push Ups, with greater load placed on working musculature due to the angle.

Key Points: Same as Push Ups above. The less leg/foot on the ball, the more difficult the exercise becomes.

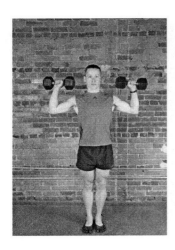 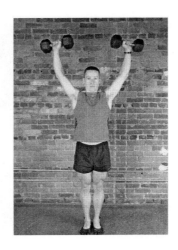

SHOULDER PRESS

Benefits: Strengthens shoulders and triceps in a motion which begins to resemble the SWIMMING motion.

Key Points: Do not hyperextend lumbar spine in order to lift the weight. Never press from behind the neck.

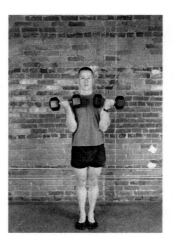 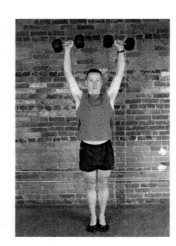

Benefits: Same as Shoulder Press above.

Key Points: Same as Shoulder Press above.

ARNIE PRESS

193

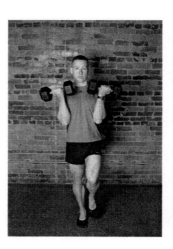 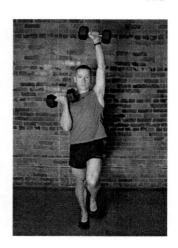

Benefits: Same as Arnie Press above with greater transfer-of-training effect as unilateral aspect more   UNILATERAL ARNIE PRESS
closely resembles SWIMMING.

Key Points: Take dominant leg away first.

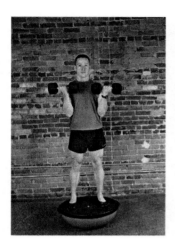 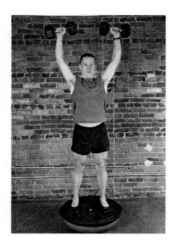

BOSU ARNIE PRESS

Benefits: Same as Arnie Press above with greater requirement to balance and utilize core and stabilizer musculature.

Key Points: Same as Arnie Press above. Utilize one leg as proficiency allows.

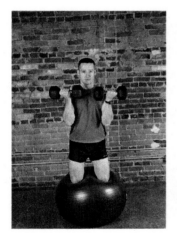 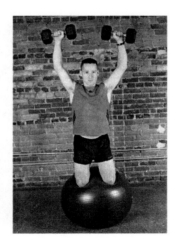

KNEELING-ON-PHYSIO-BALL ARNIE PRESS

Benefits: Same as Bosu Arnie Press above with an advanced demand for balance, core, and stabilizer proficiency due to the mobility of the ball.

Key Points: Maintain perfect posture throughout.

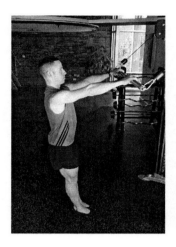
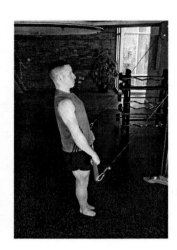

Benefits: Strengthen the latissimus dorsi, triceps, and abdominals as they stabilize against the force generated by the lats in a motion which resembles the propulsive phase of SWIMMING.

Key Points: Do not allow the thoracic spine to flex forward.

STRAIGHT-ARM
PUSH DOWNS

195

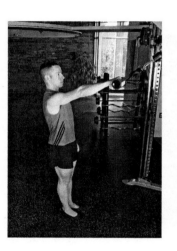

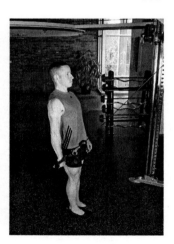

Benefits: Same as Straight-Arm Push Down above but with greater stabilizer/neutralizer activation and higher degree of strength transfer due to unilateral component.

Key Points: Same as Straight-Arm Push Down above.

UNILATERAL STRAIGHT-
ARM PUSH DOWNS

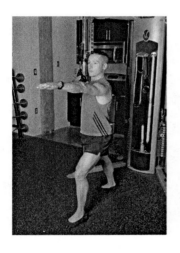 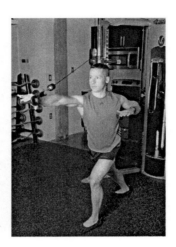

CABLE PUSH

Benefits: Integrates trunk and arm movement while improving core stabilization.

Key Points: Maintain perfect spinal/postural alignment. Movement emanates from core—do **not** push using just the arm. Handle stops at end range of motion during shoulder abduction—do **not** allow handle to go behind shoulder.

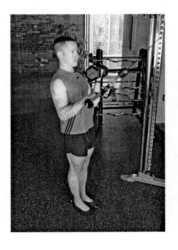 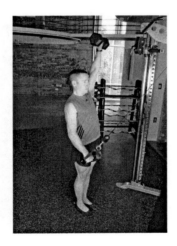

SWIM

Benefits: Trains the push pattern with high transfer of training to the SWIM.

Key Points: Keep TVA activated so pelvis doesn't deviate from underneath the shoulders.

Leg Manipulations

85% of gait takes place on one leg. Thus, doing any of the above exercises on one leg increases the difficulty of the movement while providing greater transfer of training to the sport of triathlon.

Benefits: Minimizing the base of support ramps up neural drive and the requirement for core control as well as more closely resembling the unilateral aspect of sport.

Key Points: Begin with non-dominant leg.

Varied stances (ordered from least difficult to most difficult):

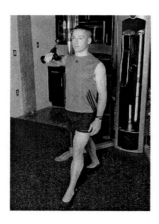

COUNTER STANCE

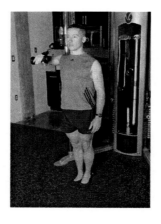

PARALLEL STANCE

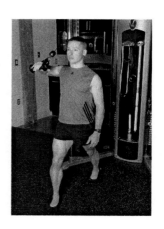

IPSILATERAL STANCE

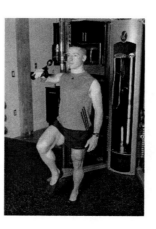

SINGLE LEG CONTRALATERAL

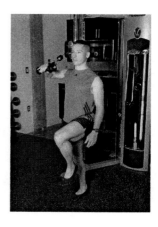

SINGLE LEG IPSILATERAL

BEND

One of the most important of the primal patterns, this movement is one we perform multiple times a day without much thought. It's probably not on our mind when we're bent over the bars during the bike leg of a triathlon either. But we stand up and take notice when we realize that strength in this pattern helps us actually to be *straight* when we stand up! Bending strengthens both the ligamentous system and the muscular system, without which we'll be running out of T2 folded at the waist. Thus, this movement pattern is critical. If the triathlete can't bend, he'll break.

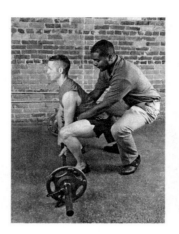
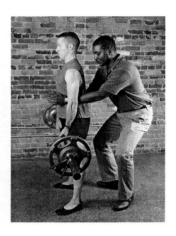

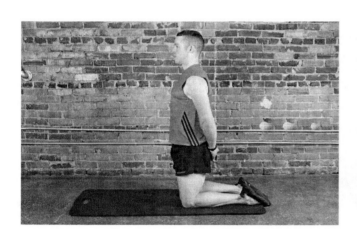
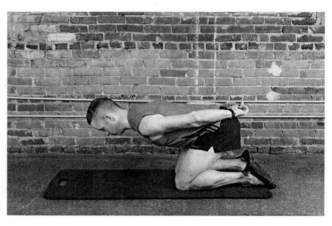

SECOND DESCENT—FROM KNEES

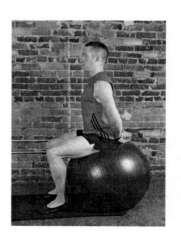
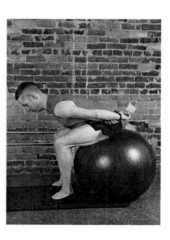

THIRD DESCENT—FROM SEATED

EXAMPLE EXERCISES

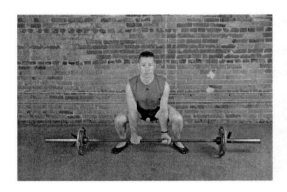 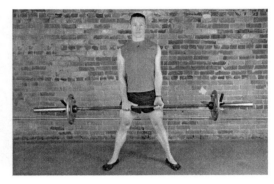

DEAD LIFT

Benefits: Strengthens legs and back.

Key Points: Maintain TVA activation and do not allow back to round into kyphosis or shoulders to protract. Head should be held in a neutral position. Release air through pursed lips as you pass through the sticking point. Knees should track over toes.

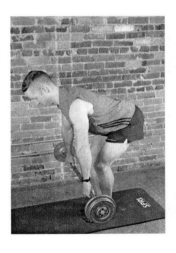 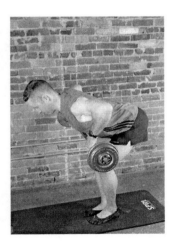

BENT-OVER ROW

Benefits: Strengthens external shoulder rotators with emphasis on development of muscular endurance of lumbar spine, which is crucial in maintenance of hydrodynamic position during the SWIM, aero position during the BIKE, and erect posture during the RUN.

Key Points: Maintain lordosis, high elbows, and TVA activation throughout movement. Keep head aligned with rest of spine so as not to perpetuate shortening of the suboccipitals which occurs through CYCLING

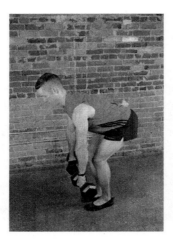 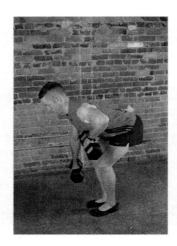 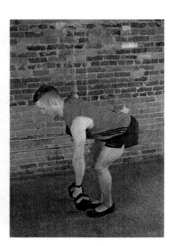

Benefits: Same as Bent-Over Row above in a unilateral environment which more closely resembles the **ALTERNATING UNILATERAL** demands of SWIMMING and RUNNING as well as out-of-the-saddle climbing on the BIKE. **BENT-OVER ROW**

Key Points: Maintain palm in, lordosis, and TVA activation throughout movement. Like Bent-Over Row above, keep head aligned with rest of spine.

201

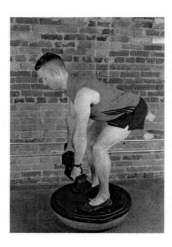 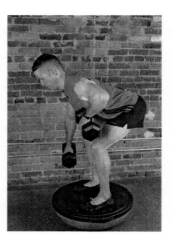 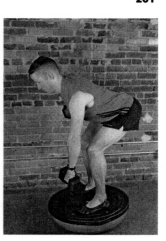

Benefits: Same as Alternating Unilateral Bent-Over Row above but on an unstable surface, requiring **ALTERNATING UNILATERAL** more core control, balance, and neural excitation. **BENT-OVER ROW ON BOSU**

Key Points: Same as Alternating Unilateral Bent-Over Row above.

NOTE: The following exercises are the ones which should be utilized when the training program calls for "back extension" movements.

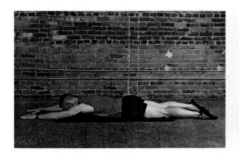 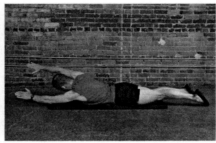 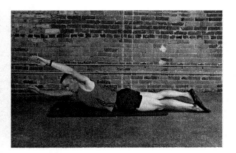

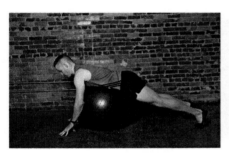 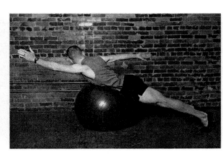 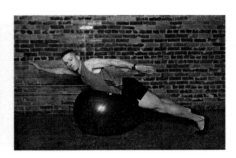

TWISTING BACK-EXTENSION (ON BALL)	**Benefits:** Strengthens the extensor chain with an emphasis on the transverse plane. Movement resembles the rotational aspect of the SWIM.
	Key Points: Do not hyperextend spine as this can irritate the facet joints and cause inhibition of the multifidus and the other muscles of the Inner Unit.

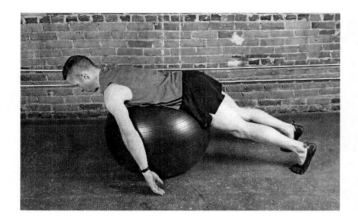
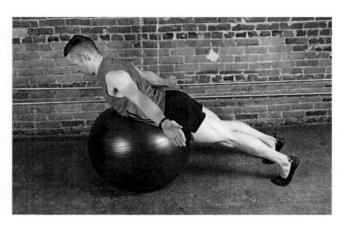

Benefits: Strengthens key postural muscles while correcting forward head posture and thoracic kyphosis.   PRONE COBRA ON BALL

Key Points: Hold head in neutral alignment at all times. Activate the glutes if exerciser has hyperlordosis of lumbar spine. If lumbar curvature is not sufficient, keep glutes relaxed to allow lumbar erectors to work.

203

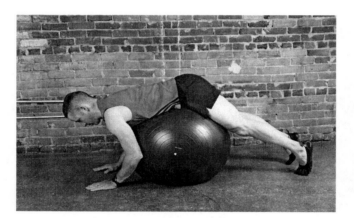
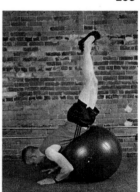

Benefits: Strengthens the extensor chain with the torso anchored such that the legs must be   REVERSE HYPER-
elevated. This aids in the ability to keep the legs in the same horizontal plane as the rest of the body   EXTENSION ON BALL
during SWIMMING.

Key Points: Focus on lifting the legs with the gluteals.

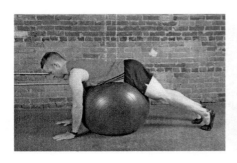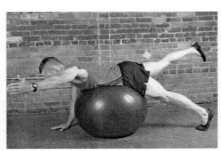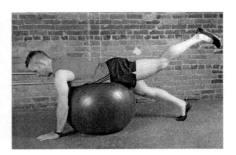

ALTERNATING SUPERMAN ON BALL	**Benefits:** Strengthen back stabilizers, including muscles like the multifidus which may be difficult for the athlete to activate consciously. The unstable aspect of the Swiss Ball is seen as threatening by the brain, allowing it to activate muscles which may have previously been inhibited.
	Key Points: Arms should come out at 45° from the body and lead with the thumbs. Maintain activation of the TVA and do not hyperextend spine.

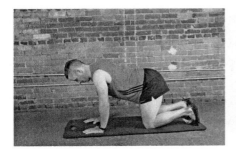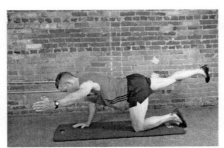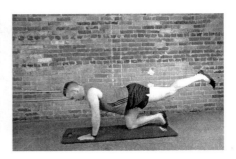

HORSE STANCES (HORIZONTAL SHOWN)	**Benefits:** Activates the small stabilizer muscles of the spine, specifically the multifidi, while strengthening key postural muscles. Training the muscles of the posterior thigh helps to maintain balance in the musculature of the legs.
	Key Points: Maintain TVA activation and neutral spinal curvatures throughout. A dowel rod may be used for cueing.

TWIST

Usually coupled with other movements, twisting is an integral part of most sports, and triathlon is no exception. In fact, rotation is the core of all movement. Swimming is predicated on rotation. If a runner can't twist, the movements which propel him forward are not only shortened, they are less efficient and the restriction will likely cause a compensation which will result in injury. Even cycling has rotational forces which must be stabilized in the body to deliver optimal power to the pedals. Proficiency in the twist pattern, then, should be a goal of every triathlete who wants to make it, not only to the starting line, but to the finish line as well.

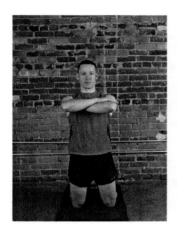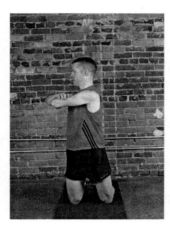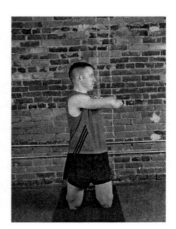

FIRST DESCENT—KNEELING

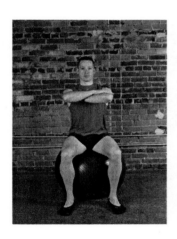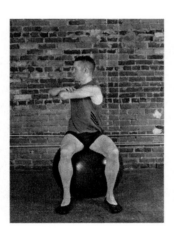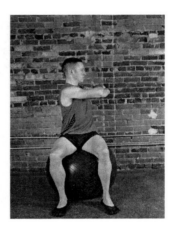

SECOND DESCENT—SEATED ON SWISS BALL

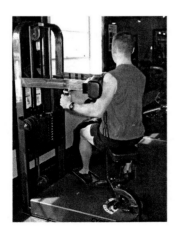

THIRD DESCENT—SEATED ON MACHINE

EXAMPLE EXERCISES

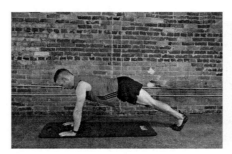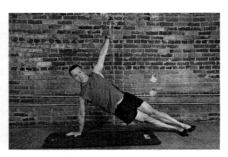

Benefits: Trains the twist pattern with minimal loading of the axial skeleton.

Key Points: Maintain neutral spinal curvatures throughout movement. Descend the exercise to just the rotational component with no push up if form necessitates making the movement easier. Moving feet closer together minimizes base of support and increases the difficulty of the exercise.

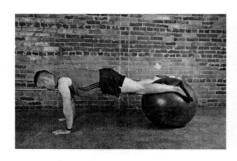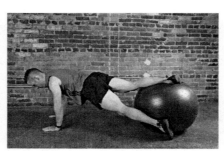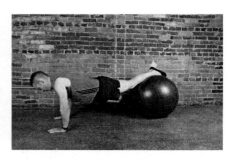

Benefits: Trains the twist pattern with the hands fixed as they should be when SWIMMING.

Key Points: Maintain TVA activation and neutral spinal curvatures throughout.

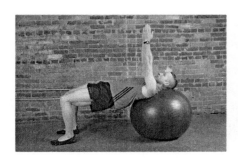 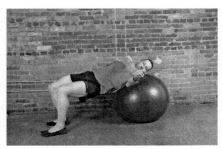 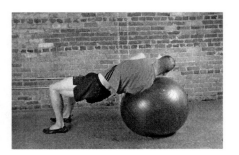

UPPER-BODY
RUSSIAN TWISTS

Benefits: Strengthen the hip extensors as well as countless muscles involved in transverse-plane motion.

Key Points: Keep tongue in *physiological resting position*, which is on the roof of the mouth behind the teeth. This position can be easily found by swallowing—where the tongue ends up is the proper position.

Holding the tongue in this position is important any time the head is held up against gravity (as in a crunch). This will activate the infra- and suprahyoid muscles. Failure to do so will necessitate using only the sternocleidomastoid (SCM) muscles and deep cervical flexors to lift the weight of the head, causing hypertrophy of these muscles as well as atrophy of the infra- and suprahyoids. Since the SCM is an extensor of the lower cervical spine and a flexor of the upper cervical spine, this muscular imbalance leads to a forward head posture and possibly hypertonicity and pains in the neck as the deep cervical flexors become overworked.

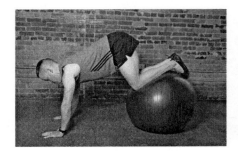 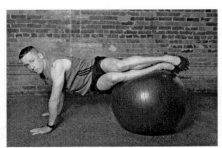 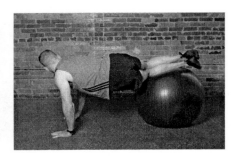

LOWER-BODY
RUSSIAN TWISTS

Benefits: Trains the twist pattern with the hands fixed as they should be when SWIMMING.

Key Points: Maintain TVA activation throughout.

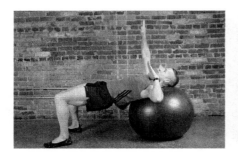 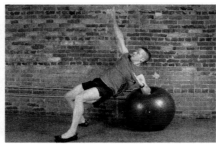 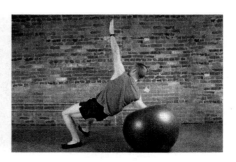

Benefits: Integrates upper and lower extremities in an explosive rotational movement as is characteristic **DROP AND RECOVER**
of triathlon, with requirements for both dynamic and static stability.

Key Points: Do not allow elbow to collapse toward body when pushing into ball.

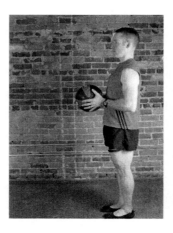 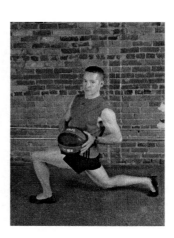

Benefits: Same as Lunge Walk above with an added rotary component as is encountered during **TWISTING LUNGE (WALK)**
RUNNING. Teaches the lower extremities to resist the frontal- and transverse-plane forces incurred during
RUNNING so key joints track properly and maintain ideal alignment.

Key Points: Twist toward the forward leg. Maintain upright posture at all times.

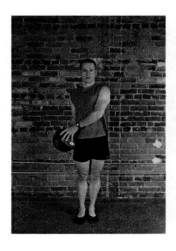 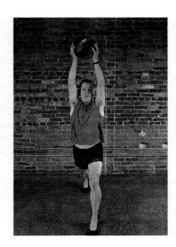 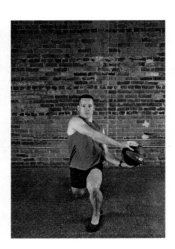

LUNGE (WALK) ARC

Benefits: Same as Twisting Lunge above with heightened neural excitation due to integration of upper-body movement.

Key Points: Arc to the side you are stepping and utilize core to keep torso from side bending with the medicine ball.

ABDOMINAL-SPECIFIC MOVEMENTS

Because the faulty head position is usually compensatory to a thoracic kyphosis, which in turn may result from postural deviations of the low back or pelvis, it is frequently necessary to begin treatment by correction of the associated faults. Treatment for the neck may need to begin with exercises to strengthen the lower abdominal muscles...

—Florence Kendall

EXAMPLE EXERCISES

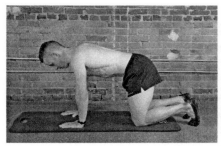 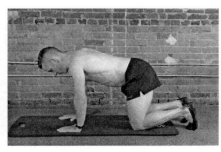 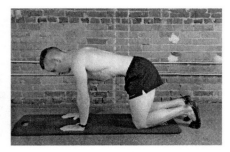

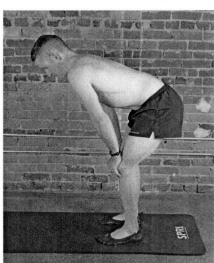 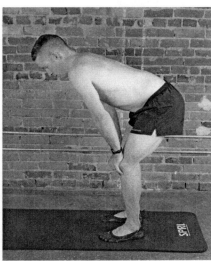 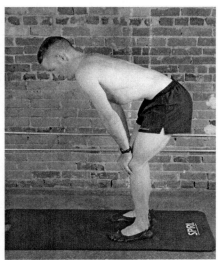

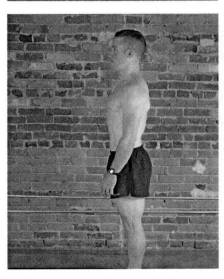 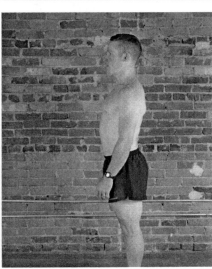 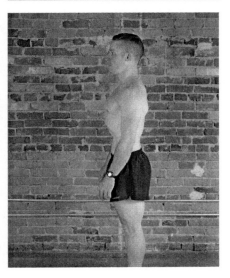

FOUR-POINT TVA STANCE AND PROGRESSIONS

Benefits: Learn how to activate the TVA. Four-point stance facilitates the learning process as the weight of the viscera puts the abdominal wall on stretch, thus increasing neural awareness of the TVA.

Key Points: Take a diaphragmatic breath before drawing your navel toward your spine. There should be no movement of the lumbar spine. Do not hold your breath

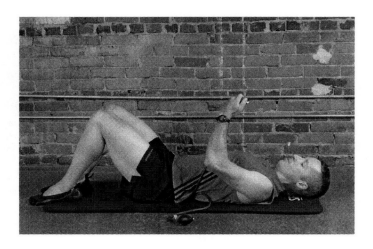

Benefits: Establishes neuromuscular control of lower abdominals while integrating TVA activation and pelvic stabilization.

Key Points: Draw umbilicus in slightly before performing posterior pelvic tilt to flatten lumbar spine against hand or blood pressure cuff and keep hamstrings relaxed.

LOWER ABDOMINAL
SERIES # 1—PELVIC TILT

213

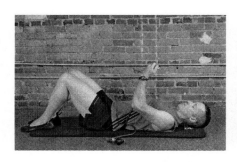 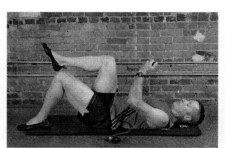 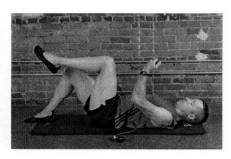

Benefits: Integrate movement into neural control of the lower abdominals.

Key Points: Activate TVA before rotating pelvis posteriorly to flatten lumbar spine. Lift one foot off floor until thigh is perpendicular to floor while maintaining constant pressure of lumbar spine against hand or blood-pressure cuff, alternating sides.

LOWER ABDOMINAL
SERIES #2A

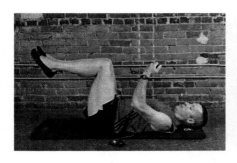 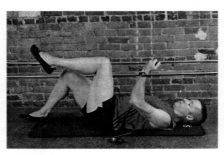 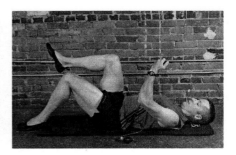

LOWER ABDOMINAL SERIES #2B

Benefits: Same as Lower Abdominal #2A above but with increased loading of the lower abdominals as start position is with feet elevated.

Key Points: Same as Lower Abdominal #2A above.

NOTE: All of the Lower Abdominal Series are best performed with a blood-pressure cuff placed opposite the navel and inflated to 40 mmHg (or 30 mmHg if lumbar curvature is deficient). The athlete would then increase the reading on the dial 30 mmHg by posteriorly rotating the pelvis to increase the pressure. For Lower Abdominal #2A and #2B, the leg movements should be performed with no more than 5 mmHg fluctuations above or below starting pressure (i.e., 60 or 70 mmHg).

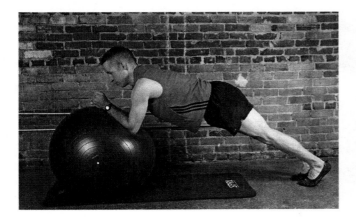 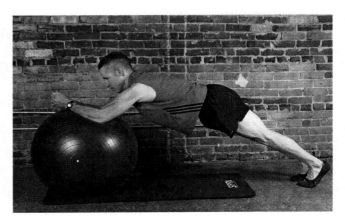

FORWARD BALL ROLL

Benefits: Strengthens abdominals against pull of latissimus dorsi (as is necessary in SWIMMING). Improves spinal stabilization while training the deep abdominal wall.

Key Points: Maintain neutral lumbar curvatures at all times. Abdominals should increase activation as ball moves away from body—do not fire abdominals maximally from the beginning of the exercise.

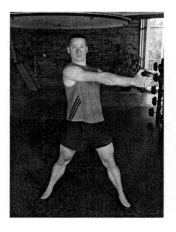 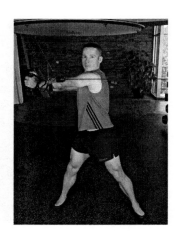

Benefits: Trains the twist pattern from a functional, standing position.

OBLIQUE CABLE TWIST

Key Points: Movement begins at the core. Rotate along the axis of your spine, trying to avoid both flexion and extension.

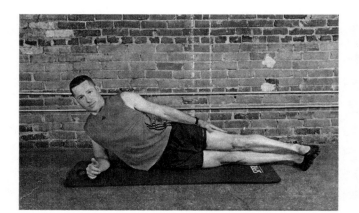 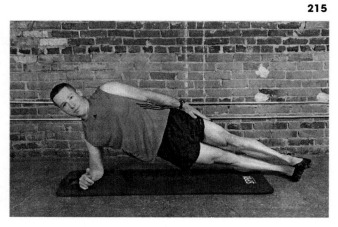

Benefits: Trains pelvic stabilization in the frontal plane.

OBLIQUE RAISE

Key Points: Draw umbilicus inward before initiating movement and do not allow body to fall out of the frontal plane.

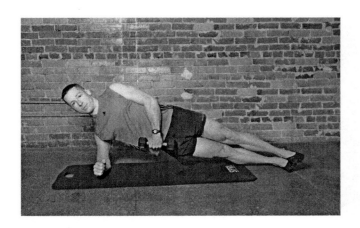 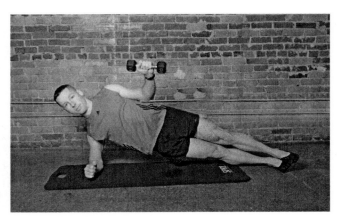

OBLIQUE RAISE EXTERNAL SHOULDER ROTATION

Benefits: Same as Oblique Raise above with additional emphasis on strengthening the external shoulder rotators with arm movement.

Key Points: Same as Oblique Raise above.

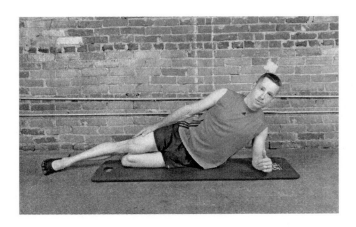 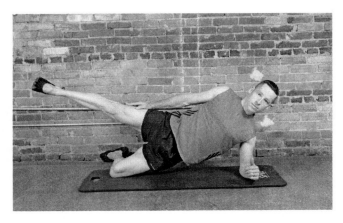

OBLIQUE RAISE ABDUCTOR

Benefits: Same as Oblique Raise above with additional emphasis on glute medius strengthening with leg movement.

Key Points: Same as Oblique Raise above.

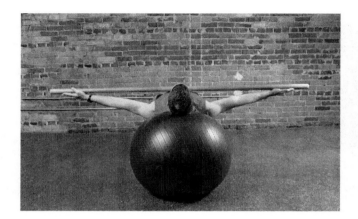
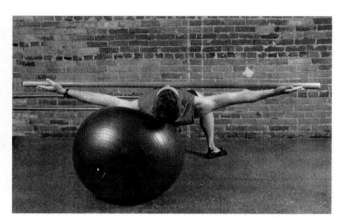

Benefits: Conditions in all planes of motion with integration of upper and lower body.

Key Points: Tongue on roof of mouth behind teeth (physiological rest position).

SUPINE LATERAL
BALL ROLL

217

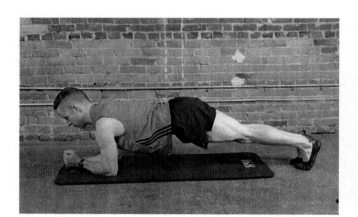
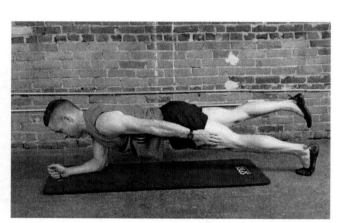

Benefits: Strengthens core musculature in a static position with additional development of upper and lower extremities, dependent on the variation employed.

Key Points: Maintain neutral spinal curvatures. If lower back begins to be the focus of the effort rather than the abdominals, stop the movement before fatigue forces form failure.

STABILIZER SERIES

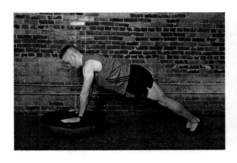 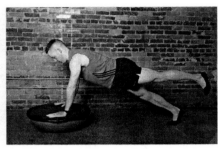 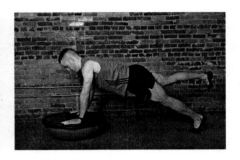

BOSU PRONE LEG LIFT

Benefits: Strengths core musculature in a static position with additional emphasis on lateral stability as a diagonal force must be controlled to maintain neutral spinal curvatures.

Key Points: Same as Stabilizer Series above. Include a push up with the movement as proficiency/posture allows.

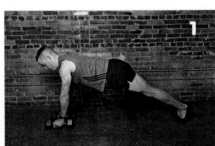 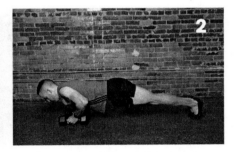

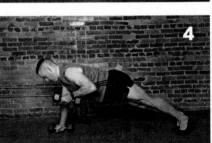 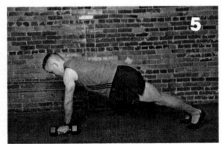

PUSH UP ROW

Benefits: Same as Bosu Prone Leg Lift above.

Key Points: Same as Stabilizer Series above. Eliminate the push up portion of the movement if form is deficient.

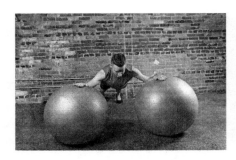 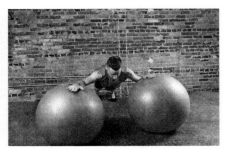

Benefits: Trains core stability while integrating arm movement with a motion similar to SWIMMING.

Key Points: Activate TVA and hold spine in neutral position.

PRONE LOW CRAWLER

219

NON-AXIAL-LOADING LEG MOVEMENTS

EXAMPLE EXERCISES

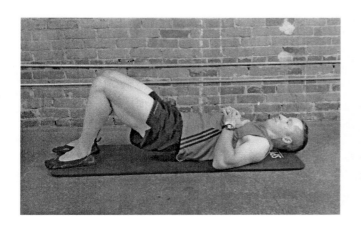 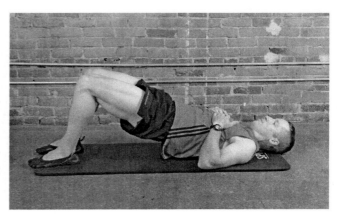

SUPINE HIP-EXTENSION

Benefits: Strengthens the hamstrings, glutes, and lumbar erectors.

Key Points: Push through heels to activate glutes. Effort should not be felt in quads. Maintain TVA activation to eliminate hyperextension of lumbar spine.

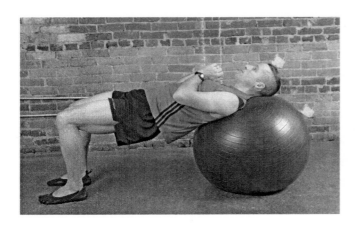 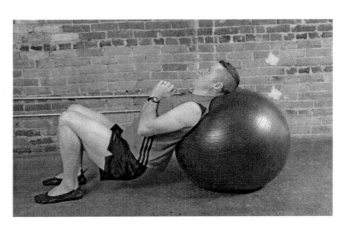

SUPINE HIP-EXTENSION

BACK ON BALL

Benefits: Strengthens the hamstrings, glutes, and lumbar erectors in an unstable, three-dimensional environment.

Key Points: Same as Supine Hip-Extension above. Move up/down, not fore/aft.

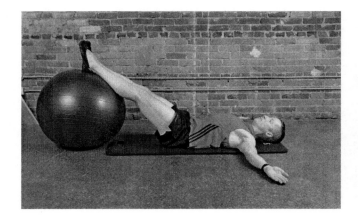
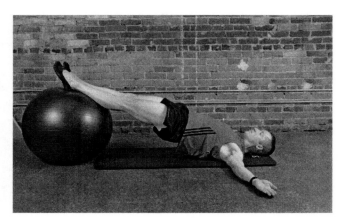

Benefits: Same as Supine Hip-Extension Back on Ball above.

Key Points: Same as Supine Hip-Extension Back on Ball above. Palms up.

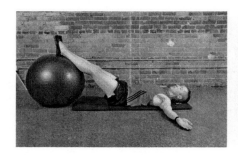
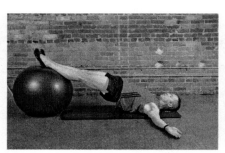
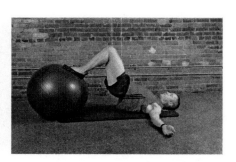

Benefits: Strengthens and integrates hamstrings, glutes, and lumbar erectors in an unstable, three-dimensional environment while improving knee stability.

Key Points: Same as Supine Hip-Extension Feet on Ball above.

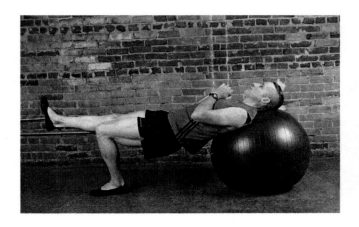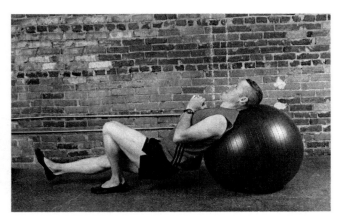

UNILATERAL SUPINE
HIP-EXTENSION
BACK ON BALL

Benefits: Unilateral position more closely resembles demands of BIKE/RUN.

Key Points: Same as Supine Hip-Extension Back on Ball above.

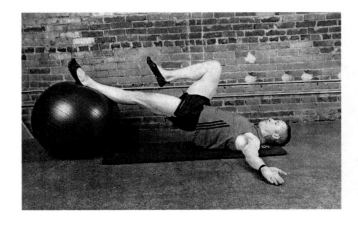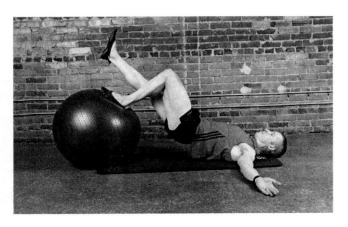

UNILATERAL SUPINE
HIP-EXTENSION
KNEE FLEXION

Benefits: Same as Unilateral Supine Hip-Extension Back on Ball above with increased neural activation of hamstring and gastrocnemius.

Key Points: Same as Supine Hip-Extension Feet on Ball above. Keep pelvis square.

Detailed descriptions of all the exercises listed above can be found on the author's website: **www.triumphtraining.com**

THE POWER OF PUTTING IT ALL TOGETHER

CHAPTER 1:

AN EXAMPLE SEASON

October 11-31 **TRANSITION—no weight training** (3 weeks)

November 1-December 12 **ANATOMICAL ADAPTATION** (6 weeks)

December 13-January 23 **MAXIMUM STRENGTH** (6 weeks)

January 24-March 6 **POWER COMPLEXITY** (6 weeks)

March 7-April 3 **MAXIMUM STRENGTH** (4 weeks)

April 4-June 26 **STRENGTH MAINTENANCE and PREHAB AND POSTURAL CORRECTION PHASE** (alternating workouts for 12 weeks)

June 27-July 10 **TRANSITION—no weight training** (2 weeks)

July 11-July 31 **ANATOMICAL ADAPTATION** (3 weeks)

August 1-August 21 **MAXIMUM STRENGTH** (3 weeks)

August 22-September 11 **POWER COMPLEXITY** (3 weeks)

September 12-October 8 **STRENGTH MAINTENANCE and PREHAB AND POSTURAL CORRECTION PHASE** (alternating workouts for 4 weeks)

There are literally thousands of different ways to periodize strength training throughout the season. Each athlete is unique, presenting with different orthopedic limitations, physical strengths and weaknesses, and triathlon goals for a particular season. The above plan is written for a two-peak season, beginning immediately following the Big Show in Kona. The first peak is for a mid-season qualifier (Ironman Coeur d'Alene) followed by a second peak for the Hawaii Ironman World Championships in October.

A two-peak season is preferable to a season with only one peak, even if you only have one goal race on the calendar. The main reason is that a second peak will usually bring about a higher level of fitness for an athlete, assuming a proper recovery and build up after the first peak. Also, it is widely accepted that peak form can only be maintained for about six weeks. Thus, a season with two peaks gives an athlete twelve weeks to race and perform at his or her best.

In the above example, you'll notice that the phases in the second half of the season are cut in half. This is to accommodate the increased training intensity as the triathlete moves toward the second and typically more important goal for the year. Muscle memory also allows for quicker adaptation during any particular phase, necessitating a more frequent change in stimulus.

If the timing of the athlete's second goal race does not allow for three weeks in either the MS or PC phases, cutting back to two weeks per training period would be an effective solution. However, if the timing only allows for one week in each phase, I'd recommend utilizing just one specific phase of two weeks based on the athlete's admitted weakness or the biomotor demand of the targeted race. Typically, my choice would be the PC phase for all but the most mountainous of races, in which case the MS phase should be utilized. Extreme ectomorphs (tall and thin body types) and female triathletes for whom cycling is the weakest discipline should also focus on the MS phase if unable to incorporate both weight periods prior to the second goal of the season.

Recovery weeks are not highlighted in the above sample season. Failure to include adequate unloading time at regularly scheduled intervals, however, would be a critical oversight. The intensity or volume of swimming, cycling, and running during the course of the season must consistently allow for appropriate rest for the triathlete to benefit from previous training and the concept of supercompensation. So, too, should the strength-training year have planned recovery weeks during which variables are manipulated to stimulate recovery.

In the above example, I would design rest weeks to fall every third week during any three- or six-week period. In training phases four or twelve weeks in duration, I'd recommend building for three weeks and then recovering for one. Of course, your planned season will often not have such round numbers, especially if you have multiple race goals during the year. So you may best be served with four weeks up and one week down, or even five build weeks followed by one down week. I do not advise trying to extend the periods between rest weeks any longer than that, however—the longer one pushes without adequate recovery, the greater the risk of mental or physical fatigue and injury. Conversely, a one-week-up-one-week-down protocol does not efficiently progress the athlete—the gains in strength experienced are incremental at best.

The definition of rest probably needs to be clarified here. After all, triathletes are notorious for doing too much when it comes to just about everything except when it comes to the concept of recovery. So here are the parameters when it comes to strength-training down weeks in specific phases:

- In the Anatomical Adaptation Phase, cut out a set (i.e., a circuit) while maintaining all other variables (reps/weight/rest/tempo) at the same level as the last workout.

- During the Maximum Strength Phase, drop down to three sets if using a four- or five-set protocol. If employing just three sets in recent training, reducing volume to two sets would be ideal. Either way, you should also decrease the number of days devoted to strength training by one day. One final recommendation is to decrease the number of reps by two while keeping the intensity (i.e., weight) at the most recent level.

- The Power Complexity Phase follows the same guidelines as the Maximum Strength Phase above.

- During both the Strength Maintenance Phase and the Prehab and Postural Correction Phase, decrease the number of sets by one while maintaining all other variables at current levels.

227

IN SUMMARY:

- Rest every three to six weeks.

- Rest weeks consist of (dependent on the current training phase) either

  One less day devoted to resistance training

  One or two fewer sets

  Two fewer repetitions

SPECIFIC GUIDELINES FOR THE THREE WEEKS PRECEDING GOAL RACE:

- No axial-loading leg movements performed in the last twenty-one days prior to key event.

- Non-Axial-Loading Leg movements can be continued until fourteen days prior to key event.

- No arm movements performed in the last ten to fourteen days before key event (unless goal race is a duathlon—then seven days should be the cutoff).

- Drill and Core work can be continued through the week of the key event at intensities and volumes which do not elicit soreness or detract from quality of swim/bike/run training.

CHAPTER 2:

WORKING IN vs. WORKING OUT

The body thrives off homeostasis. When pushed out of this state of equilibrium, just like a person who unexpectedly trips, it will quickly try to right itself. Yet trying to balance the body's billions of chemical processes that take place every second is no easy task. Making this feat even more difficult is the fact that everybody has their own specific set point for any particular physiological marker. For example, the average body temperature is 98.6° Fahrenheit. But that's an *average*. Some people naturally run hotter, while others' normal body temperature is a bit cooler. What's more, these unique parameters can fluctuate in response to a variety of internal and external factors. Thus, what is healthy for one person may not be healthy for another person or that same person at a different time.

Applied to the triathlete, this concept dictates how much training an individual can absorb. Too little, and the stimulus is not sufficient to force the body to adapt and improve. Too much, and the system becomes overly taxed. The intelligent triathlete will honor the body with rest and reap the rewards of supercompensation, while his less-perceptive counterpart will continue to ignore the warning signs until his system revolts.

Genetics and experience as well as age and health status all affect an individual's threshold for the stress of training. And make no mistake about it; training is a stress on the body. The error most triathletes make is they don't realize that the body does not differentiate between one stressor and another. As far as the body is concerned, stress is stress.

Have you ever faced a long day at work when you were under constant pressure to meet a deadline? So you wake up early, skip breakfast, fight rush-hour traffic, have lunch at the vending machine, forget to drink anything other than the coffee you spill on your shirt, misplace an important file, and get yelled at by your boss. Then, to blow off some steam, you go out for a run as soon as you get home and unwittingly add fuel to the flame. As far as your body is concerned, you just completed a ten-hour race. So that thirty-minute jog ends up pushing your tachometer into the red. You feel like crap during the whole run and crawl back home convinced you're out of shape. The big race is coming up, so you decide to set the alarm an hour earlier to get in a workout before work. You have trouble sleeping and are just nodding off when the alarm rings at 4:30 a.m. After slogging through a master's swim, you decide you need to drop some weight. So you throw back a low-calorie

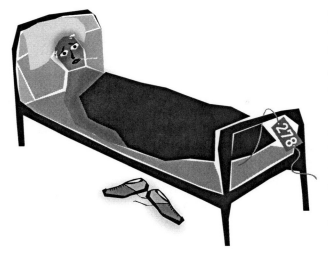

protein shake for lunch while on a conference call at your desk and hope you can keep from nodding off before quitting time. Then your bike ride after work gets delayed because your wife asks you to pick the kids up from soccer practice. When you finally get on the trainer, it's 9 p.m. and you're exhausted. The workout doesn't do much for your fitness, but it does get you wired. As you lie awake in bed, you notice a familiar tickle in the back of your throat—which always means you're getting a cold.

There goes another week of training.

Yet, the more important thing you've lost is homeostasis. More specifically, the two parts of your autonomic nervous system, the **parasympathetic nervous system** and your **sympathetic nervous system** are out of balance. The parasympathetic nervous system (PNS) is the branch of your autonomic nervous system which controls repair as well as digestion and elimination. Often called the anabolic nervous system, it stimulates the immune system and is in charge of key substances in rebuilding the body such as growth hormone, testosterone, and dehydroepiandrosterone (DHEA). The sympathetic nervous system (SNS), which produces the glucocorticoids adrenaline (or epinephrine) and cortisol, is also referred to as the "fight or flight" nervous system. Activated any time energy is needed to face or escape danger, it shunts blood away from the organs of the body and into the muscles to prepare for action.

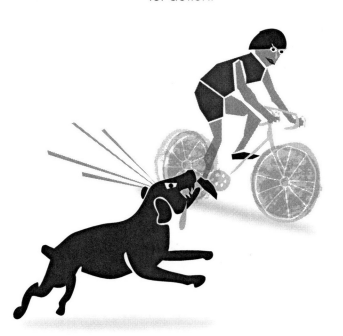

I remember a training ride I was on when I lived in Spain. I was doing hill repeats on a steep climb about ten kilometers long. My plan called for five efforts that day, and I was cranking them out as hard as I could.

Or so I thought.

About three-fourths up the climb on my last repeat of the day, a big dog rushed out of nowhere, growling and running straight at my legs. I jumped on the pedals and let out a guttural roar of instinct. Jaws closed on my foot, which slipped out of his bite as he snapped the air. His breathless growls merged with my own as I shot up the hill, the sound of his claws on the pavement disappearing behind me.

It was my fastest climb of the day.

So the action for which the SNS prepares the body obviously includes cycling. Thankfully! Indeed, it is the dominant branch of the autonomic nervous system during swimming and running, too. So anytime you're training for or competing in a triathlon, you are turning on the SNS. And if you could position a ferocious dog out on the course whenever you needed a boost, you could jack up the SNS's contribution to your race performance. To have the race of your life, you could, literally, race for your life. But I wouldn't recommend doing that frequently.

The SNS is the catabolic or tissue-destroying system, and is the yang to the yin of the PNS. When the SNS is dominant, the PNS is inhibited. That's one reason why it's so hard to eat in a race environment. The harder an athlete goes, the more the PNS and, thus, digestion becomes impaired.

Think about it. If you're running for your life, which in the era of our ancestors (before anyone had ever even heard of triathlons) is basically the only time a person would run for hours at a time, blood flow to aid in digestion takes a back seat to blood flow to fuel your legs and get the hell out of Dodge. If your body doesn't impair your digestion, it very well may end up enhancing the digestion of whatever's chasing you.

233

SNS dominance is also the explanation for the long Port-o-let lines at triathlons. Everyone's SNS is about to be ramped up, so the body gets rid of anything in the bowels which would divide the body's limited resources to eliminate. And you thought it was just the coffee...

The problem is—what if the SNS is the dominant system 24/7? What if you're that overworked, overstressed triathlete who ignores the body's growing pleas to take a break? Your PNS never gets a chance to fulfill its role of digestion and repair. You are constantly in fight or flight. You are always mobilizing and spending the body's limited resources. Your body's reserves are taxed because your digestion is impaired and you're eating processed food which is nutritionally void. You're never repairing. You're never recovering—not just from triathlon but from life, as well!

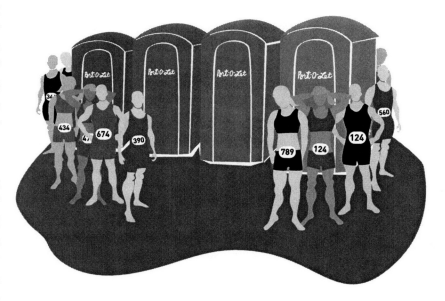

- Impaired digestion

- Impaired cognitive function

- Poor sleep quality/waking up tired

- Increased susceptibility to illness

- Constipation

- Increased respiration

- Increased heart rate

- Increased inflammation

- Increased muscle tension

- Increased abdominal fat

This is an abbreviated list of symptoms which indicate you may be suffering from an imbalance of SNS dominance in relation to the PNS. While any one specific marker is cause enough for suspicion, multiple complaints are a clear indication that you are sympathetically overloaded and the body is out of balance. The etiology of the stress could be anything—from chemical to thermal to nutritional to emotional. Yet, since all stress summates, whatever the athlete can do to curtail the cumulative impact of his or her lifestyle choices will aid in bringing the athlete back below their individual threshold or breaking point.

I purposefully use the term "breaking point" for a reason. Compared to intermittent glucocorticoid production, which has been shown to increase immunity, chronic stress begins innocently enough with an innocuous decline in physical and mental performance. Left unchecked, however, it can progress all the way to disease and even death.

In his book entitled *Why Zebras Don't Get Ulcers*, Dr. Robert M. Sapolsky's description of the Pacific salmon's life cycle is illuminating. Born in freshwater streams, the salmon migrate to the ocean before swimming thousands of miles, against the current and up waterfalls, back to their native waters to spawn. It's an arduous journey fraught with peril and requiring incredible effort. But the strongest fish eventually overcome these impossible odds and return in a miraculous display of natural instinct to the very place they were born.

Then they die.

Sort of anti-climatic, I know. And even if you're a sub-twenty-minute Olympic distance swimmer, you're not a fish—so how does this all apply to you? Well, did you ever get sick after your key event of the year? Or worse, did you catch a cold during the taper so you couldn't even make it to the starting line healthy? Not only had you been swimming as if your life depended on it. But you were cycling and running like it, too. And your sympathetic nervous system was in overdrive—just like the Pacific salmon:

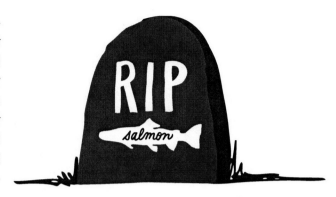

> *If you catch salmon right after they spawn, just when they are looking a little green around the gills, you find they have huge adrenal glands, peptic ulcers, and kidney lesions; their immune systems have collapsed, and they are teeming with parasites and infections.*

Yet unlike those horny little fish, you likely had to balance a nine-to-five job with family obligations, chores around the house, and the essential albeit infrequent shower. The Pacific salmon's thousand-mile journey to spawn sounds like a vacation to you. And it warrants further consideration of what chronic stress does to the triathlete. Sapolsky continues:

> *Moreover, the salmon have stupendously high glucocorticoid concentrations in their bloodstreams. When salmon spawn, regulation of their glucocorticoid secretion breaks down. Basically, the brain loses its ability to measure accurately the quantities of circulating hormones and keeps sending a signal to the adrenals to secrete more of them. Lots of glucocorticoids can certainly bring about all those diseases with which the salmon are festering.*

It's estimated that as many as 90% of the symptoms for which medical intervention is sought are related to stress and excess glucocorticoid (i.e., cortisol) production. And the minor health complaints which I listed above are just the early warning signs. Chronic stress has been shown to contribute eventually to a number of serious illnesses including:

- depression

- diabetes

- heart disease

- hyperthyroidism

- obesity

- obsessive-compulsive or anxiety disorder

- sexual dysfunction

- tooth and gum disease

- ulcers

Even cancer, which in the year 2000 was statistically reported to affect one out of every two people in the US, is affected by stress. Cortisol and the other stress hormones cause the overproduction of pro-inflammatory cytokines, as well as inhibition of the immune response to abnormal cells which would normally be destroyed before cancer had a chance to develop. So the idea that chronic stimulation of the sympathetic nervous system can actually kill seems not so far fetched. As Sapolsky writes, "Is this glucocorticoid excess really responsible for their death? Yep. Take a salmon right after spawning, remove its adrenals, and it will live for a year afterward."

Now, you *could* opt to excise your adrenals, too. But that's probably not the most practical solution. The answer for the triathlete then is to minimize every possible sympathetic stimulator so the body has more reserves to devote to coping with the stress of training. Yet sometimes, even in the best of situations, the only stressor over which the triathlete seems to have control is working out. In this case, the answer becomes simple—work in!

In contrast to working out, when a person is actually taking energy and resources *away* from the body, working in is any activity which helps increase the vitality of an individual. Examples include tai chi, basic yoga, or even gentle walking. Paul Chek, in his book *How to Eat, Move, and Be Healthy*, lists a number of different movements which he refers to as Zone Exercises. All of them are extremely effective at balancing the autonomic nervous systems as they help move chi or "life force" through the body. Whatever the chosen movement, it should finish with the body feeling energized and healthier than before the activity began.

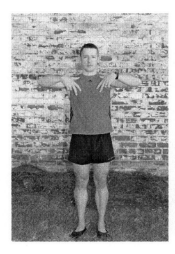 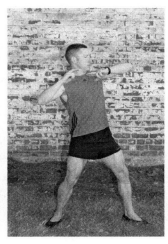 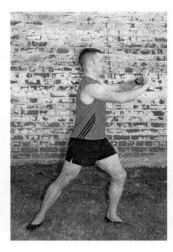 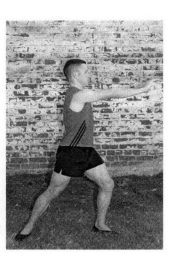

The continual contraction and relaxation of muscles involved in any exercise increases the circulation of both blood and lymph throughout the body, allowing for the removal of toxins and the mobilization of the immune system. However, when working in, the movement is performed at intensities well below that which would stimulate the sympathetic nervous system. Indeed, a good rule of thumb for some of you coming from the "more is more" philosophy of training: If you cannot comfortably perform the activity on a full stomach, you're working out, not in.

237

What about swimming, cycling, and running? Can you do any of these at "working in" intensities? Well, unless you're a 2'20" marathoner, "easy run" is an oxymoron. So running is not an option for most of us. But swimming and cycling both can be utilized to balance the autonomic nervous system if the athlete listens to his body. There should never be any muscular burn or discomfort. And you should never be out of breath. In fact, when it comes to building chi or life force in the body, you'll have more success the slower you go.

Guidelines for Working In

1. Perform at sunrise or sunset

2. Perform barefoot

3. Perform in clothing made of natural fibers

4. Perform with optimal posture

5. Perform without elevation of heart rate or respiration rate

Even if you're that rare triathlete who somehow escapes the multiple stressors with which most of us must contend on a daily basis—perhaps you live in a bubble, for example—you can still benefit by the inclusion of working-in exercises into your training program. They are ideal for your rest days, for example. Wait—you do rest, don't you? That's the biggest mistake most of my endurance athletes were making before I began coaching them. Abusing the concept of active recovery, they never truly rested enough. They weren't adequately recovered for high-intensity sessions, so their hard training became *mediocre* training. And their results became mediocre, too.

I incorporate one to two days of active recovery in my athletes' programs each week. This may range from easy sessions in the pool or on the bike, to stretching or yoga, or playing with the kids. Sometimes, complete days off are appropriate—additional training, even when easy, often equals additional stress in an already chaotic schedule—but the fitter an athlete is, the more commonly I'll prescribe some sort of movement. Otherwise, the athlete will often feel worse—clogged up and stiff. This is one reason why I'll typically eschew passive rest in favor of light activity the day before a key event. The prescribed rest day I often place two days before the race, so the athlete has a day to recover and another day to blow the exhaust out of the system.

So don't always think the answer to optimal performance can be found in training more. One of the main differences between elite amateurs and professionals is that the professional's job is his sport. So when all his training is done, he can rest while the amateur has to go to work. It really is all about recovery. Thus, oftentimes the answer lies in... well... simply lying down.

NOTE: For more information on how to perform any of the working-in movements mentioned above, please refer to the Resources Section at the end of this book.

CHAPTER 3:

NUTRITION AND LIFESTYLE CONSIDERATIONS FOR OPTIMAL PERFORMANCE

Notice this chapter isn't entitled Nutrition and Lifestyle Consideration for *Triathlon* Performance. As much as we sometimes refuse to admit it, there is life outside of triathlon. Yet current statistics might call into question the quality of that life.

- One out of three Americans is obese. Not overweight—obese!

- One out of two Americans will get some sort of cancer in their lifetime.

- Each American spends an average of $5600 a year on medical expenses.

- The US spends more money on healthcare than any other country in the world; yet we rate somewhere between 19th and 37th in the world in most major health categories.

That last bullet point begs for the question to be asked—where's that money going and why? Could it be we're looking in the wrong place for information on how to stay healthy? Last year alone *four billion* prescriptions were written by US doctors. These are the people we're going to in the name of health and fitness, yet the average life span of doctors is ten years less than for the rest of us!

Let me tell you a quick story about my former G.P. I went into his office one day. He was behind his desk as always—bent over and pale, *way* overweight and breathing hard just sitting there. He knew what I did for a living, so he goes on to tell me that he's started walking for exercise. I tell him "That's great, but I think you should also do some weight training." Then, this man who spent umpteen years in medical school so he could teach *ME* about health tells me that he doesn't want to lift weights because he doesn't want his muscles to turn to fat when he stops.

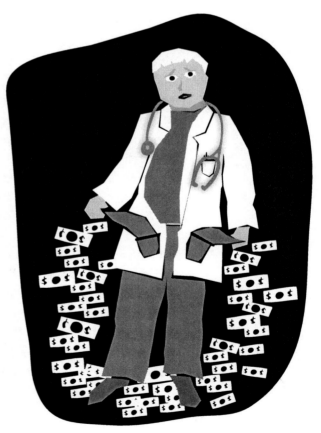

I immediately came home and told my wife, "Baby, we gotta find a new doc!"

And my new doc is awesome, so I'm not saying that all doctors are bad. I'm just saying that if your doctor smokes… or is fat… or can't walk a mile without stopping… or if he doesn't know the difference between a muscle cell and a fat cell, turn around and get the hell out of his office. At the very least, question what he's prescribing and why.

Either way, we've got to start taking responsibility for *ourselves*. We've got to stop taking health advice from those who study the sick. That's like having a financial advisor who's broke. And then there are the millions of people who listen when Oprah Winfrey tells us to rethink Kentucky Fried Chicken. The only thing we should rethink is taking advice from those who obviously aren't healthy!

We've got to get back on track! Ours isn't the first generation to lose our way. No, our parents own that dubious honor. And I know, I know… *everyone* wants to blame their parents for every emotional or spiritual issue or relationship problem we suffer from these days, but this particular distinction is justly earned. If you look at the way our grandparents lived—or, at the least, how our great-grandparents lived—it was 180° different than what we call *living* today. They might not have had all the modern conveniences we have now. But it's convenience that's killing us! Though our caloric intake has increased by more than 25% since the 1950s, our activity level has been on a steady decline, so that we are burning eight hundred fewer calories a day than we did at the start of the 20th century.

Think about it—I bet there's not one of you reading this who hasn't sat through some TV show you didn't want to watch because you couldn't find the damn remote. I've done it! *That's* convenience. And how often do you swing by the Micky D's drive-thru on the way home to pick up a Big Mac and some fries because you don't have the time or energy to make a decent meal when you get home? Convenience. Heck, you can't even find the stairs in most buildings, but the *elevator*—it's right by the front door. How *convenient*!

But we're not just eating more and moving less. We've also got *convenient* little pills for anything that ails you. Listen—I'm gonna tell you exactly what I tell my clients: A headache is not a sign you have an aspirin deficiency in your body! But we're popping pills because we're tired; we're popping pills because we can't sleep. We've got pills to save us from depression or obesity, yet we're sadder and fatter than we've ever been. We've got a pocket full of pills for all of our problems—from our incontinence to our irritable bowels to our impotence—well, not *my* impotence.

We buy over a million dollars worth of laxatives a DAY in this country. So it's not just the politicians that are full of crap! And, remember, you're not only what you eat. You're also what you don't *eliminate!*

Then you have 20% of American fifth-graders on Ritalin. That's the answer! Don't take the TV away or the Nintendo or the Frosted Flakes or the three cans of soda the average kid drinks a day. Don't worry about the 170 pounds of sugar we eat each year. Don't consider the 150 pounds of food additives. If you're like most Americans, you could probably go to your pantry, pick out any three items at random, and find that the majority of the ingredients in them were things you couldn't pronounce. And anytime you see "artificial flavor," that's actually a code word for a number of different ingredients which occur in such small quantity that the FDA doesn't require each to be listed separately—most of which you'd need a chemistry degree and a tongue that can do back flips to pronounce. In *Fast Food Nation*, author Eric Schlossler lists the ingredients of artificial strawberry flavor as

> *amyl acetate, amyl butyrate, amyl valerate, anethol, anisyl formate, benzyl acetate, benzyl isobutyrate, butyric acid, cinnamyl isobutyrate, cinnamyl valerate, cognac essential oil, diacetyl, dipropyl ketone, ethyl acetate, ethyl amyl ketone, ethyl butyrate, ethyl cinnamate, ethyl heptanoate, ethyl heptylate, ethyl lactate, ethyl methylphenylglycidate, ethyl nitrate, ethyl propionate, ethyl valerate, heliotropin, hydroxyphenyl-2-butanone (10 percent solution in alcohol), a-ionone, isobutyl anthranilate, isobutyl butyrate, lemon essential oil, maltol, 4-methylacetophenone, methyl anthranilate, methyl benzoate, methyl cinnamate, methyl heptine carbonate, methyl naphthyl ketone, methyl salicylate, mint essential oil, neroli essential oil, nerolin, neryl isobutyrate, orris butter, phenethyl alcohol, rose, rum ether, g-undecalactone, vanillin, and solvent.*

Now, personally, I'd need a shot of Ritalin just to get through that whole list.

And here's the rub. All of those additives—in fact, *anything* you put in your mouth that you were not designed to eat—will be treated in your body like a toxin. And you know what your body does with toxins? It stores them as fat. That's right—all of these multi-syllabic words that you'd need a chemistry degree to pronounce have

243

to be filtered by your liver. And what your liver can't handle gets shuttled away as fat to keep it away from your body's essential organs.

That's how they make cows fat. Cows aren't supposed to eat grains. Cows are meant to eat grass. Feeding them grains, just like what happens to us when *we* eat grains which *we're* not really designed to eat either, makes them fat. And it makes them sick, too.

It's not rocket science! Just do what your grandparents did and live like people have done for eons. Our ancestors didn't count calories or watch their fat intake. They just ate real food—minimally processed, life-giving food that's not found in a can or a box or a plastic container.

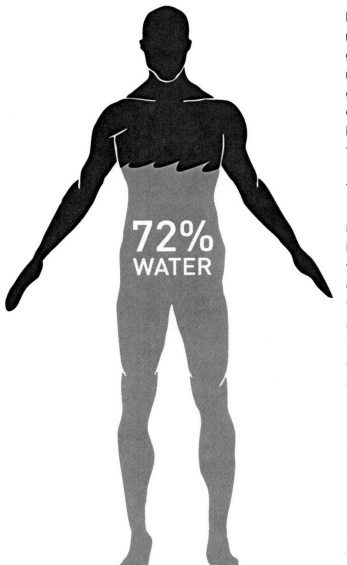

72%
WATER

It takes life to give life. So if you're eating dead, non-foods which are void of nutrition, your body's got to metabolize it somehow. It takes vitamins and minerals and protein and other micro-nutrients to get your food from mouth to anus. And if the food doesn't provide that nutrition, your body has to get it from somewhere. So it takes it from your muscles. It takes it from your bones, your ligaments, your hair!

There's a great read called *Beating the Food Giants* by Paul Stitt. He was a biochemist for a major food corporation, and his book gives startling insight into the manufacturing process of the stuff we put in our mouths. In his book, Stitt writes about an experiment his company did in which they fed a group of rats puffed-wheat cereal. Another group they fed nothing. And the last group they fed the *box* from the puffed-wheat cereal. Can you guess who died first? The rats that ate the cereal! So if you're not eating according to the rules I'll list below, your body's being forced to use your own precious tissue just to process the nutritionally void crap you're stuffing in your mouth.

And drink water, for God's sake. The body is 72% water. It's not 72% coffee or orange soda. Every physiological process in the body requires water. And we're not drinking enough.

I have a client in her sixties who started with me a little over a year ago. Now, when a person comes in to see me, the first thing I do is take them through a three-hour physical assessment. And this is after they fill out what some would say is a mountain of paperwork. Well, when I saw her walk in, I immediately called an audible. Even though my assessment's not that demanding, I could tell it'd be too much for her. She was about a hundred pounds overweight. Had 45° scoliosis, two replaced knees, was on eight different prescription meds, went to bed at 2:30 a.m., ate one meal a day, drank three cups of coffee and four diet sodas each day and, get this, only *one* eight-ounce glass of water.

So I nixed the assessment, and we just sat and talked nutrition—purely off the cuff. Within a minute she was in tears. And not because I was beating her up, but because she was a *physical* wreck. And you cannot separate the physical from the emotional from the mental from the spiritual. So I got her to focus on the positive—the fact that she was there showed she was willing to make a change—and I suggested a couple of things for her to do as "homework."

Literally a week later she came in, and I immediately saw something was different. I was thinking, "Did she lose weight? Did she get a hair cut? Something's changed." So I asked her, and she got this smirk on her face, telling me that all her friends were accusing her of having plastic surgery. Yet, all she'd done was cut out the diet drinks, gone down to one cup of coffee in the morning, and started drinking sixty ounces of water each day. And, like a giddy little school girl, she kept saying that she had all this energy now!

I know what you're saying. You're not an old lady with two replaced knees. Well, yeah, that's true—you're not... yet. And neither was the client whom I discussed in the Strength Maintenance chapter of the previous section. But she was well on her way. This gifted athlete in her twenties had become her own worst enemy. How? By training like an Olympic gold-medalist swimmer but *living* like a girl still wearing water wings in the baby pool! And she almost came to me too late. But by working on the six Foundational Principles of health briefly detailed below, we were able to bring her back from the brink of self-destruction. Not only is she an Ironwoman now, having completed Ironman Louisville in 2008; she also recently turned pro in open-water swimming and grabbed second in her first race of the year.

One of the main reasons I was inspired to write this book is that too many people believe they are immune to the impact which poor nutrition and lifestyle choices have on them, because they're triathletes. If anything, the demands of triathlon necessitate we be even more vigilant of how we treat our bodies. Even the best-designed training program will not optimize performance if the athlete's biochemistry is wrong. Exercise, especially endurance exercise, is a stress. And if you stress a system already under load, you risk breaking that system. Triathletes are the proverbial camel, with swimming, cycling, running, and weights being the straws which break their backs. The foundation for their health must be built upon more than swimming, cycling and running. It must also include instruction on proper thinking, breathing, drinking, eating, and sleep. Only then can the triathlete run the race, of multisport or of life, with the vitality essential for success.

The six Foundational Factors below can, if followed correctly, ensure the triathlete and virtually everyone enjoys a life of health and happiness.

BREATHING: It's the first thing we do when we're born, and it's the last thing we do before we die. The healthy human body can survive weeks without food and days without water. But we can only last a few minutes without oxygen. Breath *is* life force! Yet we've recently twisted the simple act of breathing into a task which directly or indirectly accounts for 70-75% of all doctor visits. We have begun to breathe exactly the opposite of how nature intended. This inverted breathing pattern creates a host of issues, from trigger points in the neck and upper back, to hormonal responses that affect literally every cell in the body. And know this: The average person breathes an amazing 25,000 times a day! This practice makes *permanent*, not perfect, so we'd better make sure we're breathing correctly.

Exercise, of course, causes an increase in respiration. Thus, the effects of faulty breathing get multiplied in the triathlete. And as the hormonal damage and postural aberrations accumulate, performance suffers in kind.

Our mouths are designed for eating, communicating, and love-making (a form of communication), not for breathing. Unless you're racing, training hard, or being chased by a sabertooth tiger, you should be breathing through your nose. This warms and filters the air. And that breath should be drawn in diaphragmatically, or into your belly. Have you ever seen a profile picture of a professional cyclist during a time trial? It may look like he has a pot belly, but he's got 4% body fat for Pete's sake. He's really just maximizing the effectiveness of each breath by breathing diaphragmatically. This helps him fill the bottom third of his lungs, where oxygen is more efficiently exchanged for carbon dioxide.

In contrast, most of us are chest breathers. We take shallow breaths in through the mouth in rapid succession. Consequently, our accessory respiratory muscles (i.e., the scalenes) become overworked, resulting in tonic painful musculature which your massage therapist just loves to find. And much like stagnant water, the air in the bottom third of the lungs becomes stale if we never replace it through proper breathing mechanics. This lack of movement (i.e., old air for new air) creates a prime breeding ground for bacteria and other pathogens. Even worse, our subconscious keeps looking for the tiger that stalked our ancestors, causing a cascade of stress hormones to circulate continuously throughout the body. And even though that tiger's really just in our subconscious, the body is innately tied to what and how we think.

THINKING is the next Foundational Factor. The average person has 60,000-70,000 thoughts running through his/her head a day. And since 80-95% of stress comes from your thoughts, it would behoove us to make those thoughts positive instead of negative. Look at someone like Natasha Badmann in her prime. The perpetual smile she had on her face, even when running through the dreaded Energy Lab of Hawaii's Big Island, should prove to you that triathlon success is more mental than physical. Heaven and hell have the same address, and the only difference between happiness and unhappiness is a *choice*. So choose to be happy. When you wake up in the morning, choose to be healthy. Think proactively, such that your life is molded by your thoughts, rather than your thoughts being manipulated by your life. Why water something you don't want to grow?

Speaking of water, **HYDRATION** is the third foundational factor critical to health. Our bodies are 72% water, and every physiological task the body performs depends on both the quality and quantity available for those processes. For example, one of the key roles water plays in the body is to aid in the elimination of the waste which gets produced in cells as a byproduct of daily functioning. The greater metabolic requirements of racing a triathlon cause the body to produce even more waste, thus necessitating even more water. The average adult has some ten trillion cells, each performing specialized functions. And if the liquids consumed only contribute to their pollution, just like mopping the floor with a bucket of dirty water, our cells remain contaminated. Health and, indeed, triathlon performance cannot thrive in such an environment.

So how much should you drink? Dr. Batmanghelidj, author of *Your Body's Many Cries for Water*, states that optimal hydration levels occur when one drinks half of his/her body weight in pounds, in ounces of water each day. So a 150-pound person would need to drink seventy-five ounces of water every day. This amount would, of course, increase with exercise or in hot climates. And if you think you can reach this daily total by dinking soda, coffee, or pasteurized juice, think again. These beverages actually contribute to dehydration as well as a host of other adverse health effects ranging from Syndrome X (i.e., insulin resistance) to tooth decay. Our bodies were meant to drink water and nothing else. Fresh-squeezed juices, in moderation, can be used judiciously by some metabolic types. And clean fuel sources like the ones sourced by Hammer Nutrition can be used when racing or training. But each of these should really be designated not as hydration but as nutrition.

247

NUTRITION is the fourth Foundational Factor. It's the inspiration for countless diet books, and entire libraries could be devoted to the misinformation continually published on this misunderstood subject. But it's so simple your grandparents could do it. In fact, our generation is probably the first which has really deviated from what our ancestors realized was common sense:

- The more ingredients in a food, the worse it is for you.

- The longer the shelf life of a food, the worse it is for you (the exceptions to the rule are raw seeds/nuts and fermented foods like sauerkraut).

- The more health claims made about a food, the worse it is for you.

- If you can't pronounce an ingredient in a food, don't eat it.

- If it hasn't been on this earth for 5000+ years, don't eat it.

- If it won't keep your dog alive, don't eat it.

- Stay away from HYDROGENATED/PARTIALLY HYDROGENATED foods (baked goods are a major culprit).

- Stay away from ARTIFICIAL COLORS/SWEETENERS/FLAVORS or PRESERVATIVES (just about anything pre-packaged).

- Eat organic/local—it's better for you, the environment, and the economy.

- Eat a balance of macro-nutrients (carbohydrate/fat/protein) at every meal/snack.

- As a general rule, color is a proxy for nutrient density in a food. If it's the color of cardboard (i.e., cereal), it probably has about the same nutritional value.

See, what we put into our mouths is recognized by the body as either a food or a toxin. Food supports and nourishes the body, allowing a miraculous array of chemical reactions to take place to run our metabolic machinery. Toxins, on the other hand, must be eliminated before they can reach dangerous levels and threaten the very survival of the body.

Of course, it takes nutrition from *real* food to "take out this trash." When these nutrients are unavailable, as so often happens from eating typical, processed-to-death *non-foods* (foods so void of nutrition that they take more from the body than they give), the body cannot get rid of these toxins. Nature has provided us, however, with an ingenious method to store these toxins safely until such factors are present that allow us to eliminate them. It's called FAT! That's right—one of fat's major roles in the body is to attract toxins and store them away from essential bodily organs. So just like a farmer fattens a cow more quickly by feeding it grains instead of grass, humans, too, get fat when we consume things we *weren't designed to eat.*

The average American eats approximately 150 pounds of carcinogenic food additives each year. Our nutrition is so poor that we could not hope to assimilate and metabolize all of the **C.R.A.P.** (**C**affeine, **R**efined sugar/flour, **A**lcohol, **P**asteurized dairy/juice), not to mention pesticides, artificial colors/flavors, and preservatives commonly found in the American diet. The result is weight gain as the body shuttles this barrage of toxins into our fat stores. Additionally, all of these processed non-foods actually rob us of nutrition: To digest this mountain of C.R.A.P., the protein, vitamins, and other essential nutrients our food should have provided are stolen from our tissues. This creates inefficient organs, weaker muscles, and brittle bones and teeth. We're literally starving to death on full stomachs! Unsatisfied on a cellular level, we're constantly hungry and looking for nutrition somewhere. The result finds more than one out of every three adults in the United States either overweight or obese. And those other two Americans? Well, they probably believe they're immune to these injustices because they belong to a gym.

EXERCISE! Is this really the panacea which will nullify the effects of a crappy diet? Well, while it may help offset some of the harm done by the two greatest weapons ever developed by man—the fork and spoon—done incorrectly, it only magnifies the dietary destruction. The two most common mistakes made by gym-goers are working muscles in isolation and exercising exclusively on machines. We've discussed the detriments of both in previous chapters. And, again, if you look at how your grandparents (or at least your great-grandparents) stayed healthy, you'll realize that papa and grandma knew more about fitness than the junk you find on the pages of some health rag, or being espoused by your average personal trainer. You would never catch either of them hammering out five sets of seated bicep curls, or destroying their knees on the leg-extension machine.

249

Some may argue that their grandparents never even worked out. But if you analyze their routine movements, you'll realize they got a "workout" every day in contrast to our largely sedentary work duties. After she woke up, grandma would probably hurry to the kitchen where she'd *squat* down to get a pan out of a cabinet, *bend* over to get meat out of the ice box, *pull* the breakfast table out of the corner, *push* chairs into place, and *twist* back and forth as she pulled utensils out of the drawer to set the table. Heck, the only movement she hadn't performed by 6 a.m. was a set of lunges!

The above actions are all primal patterns—movements which our caveman ancestors needed to be proficient in to survive. The sabertooth tiger wasn't just in their heads! If you couldn't squat, lunge, push, pull, bend, or twist, natural selection made you the best choice for that tiger's lunch! Admittedly, the modern conveniences we enjoy today have made the cost of faulty movement patterns less severe. Now the price for an inability to squat properly is the going rate for spinal surgery, which results from overusing your back. But you've got insurance—right?

The take-away message here is to get up off machines and perform compound movements which will actually lessen the likelihood of you meeting your yearly medical deductible. Use free weights and cable systems which work in all three planes of motion and don't require you to sit. Also use body-weight exercises which force you to maintain your center of gravity over your own base of support.

And if you have friends or loved ones who aren't currently working out and are really de-conditioned, just get them to perform the same activities they do daily/ weekly and take it up a notch. For example, park farther away from work or the mall or the post office or the grocery store and simply walk to the destination. Get them to work up to a minimum of twenty minutes each day. It takes energy to build energy. So simply moving more is truly an investment in themselves. As they become fitter, maybe they'll join you in this triathlon obsession. Or maybe they'll just progress to more traditional forms of exercise. But remember, a tradition is something which has been done for a while. So stay away from those machines—they're so new and unnatural that your grandparents would probably have nightmares about them.

SLEEP is the final Foundational Factor crucial to health, and one which too many triathletes commonly sacrifice. The light bulb precipitated an epidemic of sleep dysfunction from which many disease states manifest. See, our bodies are rhythmic, following predictable cycles which have become deeply ingrained in our physiology. One of these cycles is sleep. For generations, humans have gotten up with the sun and gone to bed within a few hours of sunset. Our bodies are literally designed to function on, not just a sufficient amount of sleep, but on a specific *time* for sleep, as well. The release of growth hormone and other anabolic hormones happens predominately between the hours of 10 p.m. and 2 a.m., while the second half of the sleep cycle is devoted to psychogenic repair between the hours of 2 a.m. and 6 a.m. Staying up until midnight to watch TV or work on the computer robs the body of two hours of physical recovery. Couple that with the early-morning training sessions of the typical working triathlete, and you have a recipe for more than just burnout. This error results in an inability to recover from exercise or even the activities of daily living. Aches and pains soon become chronic and the immune system weakens, allowing the body to become susceptible to pathogens from both inside and outside the body. In fact, medical professionals recognize shift work and ignoring our circadian rhythms as second only to smoking in the number and severity of adverse effects on our health. So turn off those lights.

Shut off the television. Get into bed by 10 p.m. And turn those dreams of health, and maybe even Kona, into reality.

All six of the Foundational Factors are the basis on which wellness is built; only with a solid foundation in every one of them can we build high levels of vitality and peak functioning. Of course, each of the subjects above has only been briefly introduced. For a more thorough discussion on how you can take responsibility for yourself and be in control of your own health destiny, catch me on my soapbox (which I stand on often—and not just because I'm short), read some of the works cited in the Reference List or in the Resources Section, or simply visit my website at **www.triumphtraining.com.**

THE QUESTIONS, THE ANSWERS, AND THE GLOSSARY OF TERMS

CHAPTER 1:
EPILOGUE

If I knew then what I know now.

Instructing a person on the fundamentals of proper strength training is challenging enough in a one-on-one setting. The limitations of a book make this task even more daunting. But I have done the best I can and know that the concepts contained in this work will improve both your performance and your longevity in the world of triathlon.

My life as a professional cyclist ended well before I became a strength-and-conditioning specialist. And while the skills I've gained since beginning my second career probably wouldn't have helped me avoid that last concussion, I know that this critical information would have helped me get closer to my genetic potential before I decided to hang up my wheels.

The chapters of this book are filled with over twenty years of experience as both an athlete and an exercise and rehabilitation professional. And it's the knowledge within these pages which has allowed me to compete at an elite level for many years despite a life-threatening diagnosis which has stripped me of many of my former abilities. I'm not the athlete I was. And you're not the triathlete you can be. But with continued work and this book as our guide, the only limitations we truly have are the ones we'll set for ourselves.

Questions and Answers

- ***Is there a period of the season when strength training should be emphasized over endurance training?***

We're triathletes, not weight lifters. So your sport-specific training should be emphasized for the majority of the year. The only time when strength training should be the primary focus is during the off season and during the early base-building period of your season, when intensities in all three disciplines are typically lower. This is often the time when the high-intensity strength-training phases (i.e., the MS phase and the CP phase) are incorporated into your overall program. At other times of the year, if it comes down to making a choice between a gym session or a swim/bike/run session, opt for the sport-specific one. You can (and should) still incorporate core-specific movements for five to fifteen minutes three times a week whenever you can squeeze it in.

- ***Should I stop lifting weights as I get closer to my event?***

That depends. Is it a goal race or is it just a "training" race? If it's an important event for you, then take the weights out of your program as detailed in Section Four so that you can give your body a chance to supercompensate and go into the race with fresh legs. But if it's just an event that is a step toward a bigger goal, then go ahead and train through it. I'd then advise you to schedule your last strength training day as early in the week as possible to allow for more recovery. After all, it may not be your focus for the year, but getting on the podium at a race you're not peaking for is good for the confidence level. Another alternative would be to do the second (or third) strength-training session of the week after the race. If it's a Saturday race, do your weight training on Sunday. And if it's a Sunday race—well, you know you're hardcore and getting a leg up on the competition when you're knocking out a gym session a few hours after crossing the finish line.

• How soon after a race can I resume my strength training?

Your strength training can start back up on the next scheduled session if the event wasn't too taxing. So listen to your body. It's sending you signals all the time. Most of us just ignore them; or we're so committed to following a particular training schedule that we refuse to take time off even when our bodies are demanding rest. But remember this: A muscle that's moving is a muscle that's recovering. If it's just general soreness from the race, movement will often make it feel better. Often that movement should be an easy spin or swim. But if your body and, more importantly, your mind feel recovered enough, then go ahead and do your next weight-training session as programmed. And if the first five minutes don't make you feel better than when you walked into the gym, you can either cut back on the intensity and volume for that workout or just call it a day.

• When should an athlete do his strength training? Before or after a swim, bike, or run workout or as a stand-alone training session?

The answer to that question depends on the time of the year and the current training focus of the athlete. A technique-intensive discipline like swimming or a high-intensity session in any of the three disciplines will suffer due to residual fatigue if done immediately after a weight-training session. In addition, the inherent risk of injury due to impact forces make running after weights for any considerable duration a questionable training decision. However, if enough time has passed to allow for adequate rejuvenation of the athlete's hormonal system (generally four hours or more), then a second workout should be fine and will actually facilitate recovery from the previous session.

255

Quality sessions in any of the three disciplines, typically done in the Build phase of an athlete's program (and normally corresponding with a less intense phase of weights like the SM phase) should always be done before weights or less intense swim/bike/run workouts. If strength training is scheduled for the same day, it could follow immediately for time's sake (and may well simulate the fatigue incurred during the latter stages of a race) or, ideally, several hours later. The only time when intense weight training should really be positioned as the first workout of the day is during the MS or CP phase. And these are both best followed by rest or a strictly aerobic session later in the day.

- *Are mornings or evenings better for strength training?*

From a hormonal perspective, morning sessions are always preferable for weight training as they encourage elevated levels of growth hormone as well as an increased metabolic rate for the rest of the day. Indeed, those who perform their strength-training sessions in the evening may find it difficult to sleep. That being said, quality swim, bike, or run sessions should always take precedence over weight training. But it may come down to when the athlete will do his/her strength training. Whatever that time is—morning or night—that's the best time for that athlete.

- *How about nutrition before, during, and after strength training? And what about the timing and specifics of post-training nutrition?*

Most folks just need to eat food, the definition of which can be found in Chapter Three of Section Four. But for those of you who will not be appeased until I give you some specifics, I'll make the following suggestions. I don't recommend strength training on an empty stomach. The primary source of fuel when lifting will be glycogen. So if you begin training in a fasted state, especially for workouts first thing in the morning, you risk not being able to train to your true potential. This decreased intensity will often result in a muted hormonal and metabolic response and the outcome of your time spent in the gym will be mediocre at best. If you find that eating too soon before a strength-training session leaves you feeling lethargic or in gastrointestinal distress, you need to do one of two things. Examine what you ate and think about whether or not it was appropriate for your metabolic type. Too much fat/protein can easily make you feel tired, while too many carbohydrates can have a similar effect by elevating your blood sugar too quickly, followed by an energy crash as your insulin levels rise to bring blood sugar levels back down. You may also need to push the timing of the meal back or cut down on the quantity of food so that your body doesn't remain in a parasympathetic state trying to digest what you just ate as you're trying to work out.

• *What about the saying "No pain, No gain"? Should I feel sore and stiff after my strength-training workouts?*

The saying "no pain, no gain" is responsible for numerous orthopedic and postural dysfunctions. Training should be about training, not draining. So while you should expect to be sore any time you're exposed to a new training stimulus, including a change in strength-training phases, pain and soreness should not be the goal of a particular session. It's not an indication of how effective your workout was. Rather, it's more a reflection of either how different a specific variable in the routine was compared to what you're accustomed to; or how poorly you implemented an adequate recovery strategy. You'd better hope it's not the latter.

SWIM-SPECIFIC QUESTIONS

• *No matter how hard I try, I cannot seem to improve my swim times. Are there exercises you'd suggest which might help me?*

My first suggestion is to get your stroke analyzed by a good swim coach. But you can be proactive in the meantime and focus on integrated movements with swim-specific carryover. One of my favorites would be a combination of the Bosu prone leg lift with push-up rows. It's essentially a superset of two highly effective core-focused exercises. And swimming, like all movements, starts at the core. If you're just swimming with your arms and legs, I can guarantee that you're not swimming to your potential.

257

• *I can swim with the "A" group at my master's swim class until I put a buoy between my legs. Then I get lapped at anything over a 400. What am I missing?*

Let me guess—you're a cyclist, right? You have a strong kick and probably good use of the hip extensors which have been developed over the course of hundreds or perhaps thousands of hours in the saddle. So when you put a buoy between your legs and take these muscles out of the equation, you're forced to rely on your relatively undeveloped upper body. Core movements which involve rotation would be the first place to start. I'd also employ a closed-chain movement like pull ups. And you want to make sure the triceps are strong, so a straight-arm push down or, better yet, the exercise I call the Swim would both be excellent choices.

- ***My swim starts need work. Any strength-training advice which can help me get to the front of the swim and out of the melée so that I can race the first leg of a triathlon like I know I can do?***

Short sprints on long rest as well as moderate-length efforts swum at maximum intensity for the distance should be staples in your swim workouts, especially as you near competition. But your training in the weight room could compliment this approach by using explosive movements as described in the chapter detailing the PC phase of weights. Personally, I like oblique cable twists to develop rotational power. Plyo rows and med-ball tricep throws could also be implemented, though I'd make sure the closed-chain aspect of the catch was also represented in my strength-training program by incorporating the appropriate exercise(s).

BIKE-SPECIFIC QUESTIONS

- ***I can't seem to stay in the aero position for long periods of time. What do I need to include in my strength training to address this limitation?***

The inability to maintain the aero position for extended periods of time could be related to a number of factors. Have you been properly fitted? A proper fit is essential to comfort and performance on the bike. Have you trained sufficiently in the aero position? Do you have adequate flexibility, particularly in the psoas or the hamstrings or any of the muscles in the posterior kinetic chain? If the pain is in the lower back, you may benefit from strengthening the lower abdominals. The bent-over row is another exercise which will develop postural endurance in the muscles under load when in the aero position. If the discomfort is in the neck or shoulders, an exercise like the prone cobra may be the answer.

• *I have a hard time with steep hills on the bike. Are there specific exercises you'd recommend be emphasized in my program?*

I'd first consider core strength. If it's deficient, the legs will not be able to apply power to the pedals efficiently no matter how much they can squat. Additionally, upper-body contribution is greater when out of the saddle than when seated. But if the ability to transfer the power of the arms to the legs is limited due to a weak or deconditioned core, you'll be less able to coordinate your upper-body strength with your lower-body strength.

And while an exercise like the squat is a great foundational exercise for lower-body strength, movements which are more sport-specific would be ones which focus on unilateral development. Some examples include lunges or step ups or unilateral squats. My favorite would probably be the high step up which puts the quadriceps at a mechanical disadvantage, thus necessitating the increased recruitment of the glutes and hamstrings—the powerhouses of cycling which often get neglected by quad-dominant triathletes.

You may also want to consider more complex movements that incorporate both upper-body and lower-body movements simultaneously in a cross-crawl pattern. These movements strengthen how the right and left sides of the body work together in a coordinated fashion—just like they do (or should do) on the bike.

259

• *The only time I cramp during a race is on the bike. It's always the inner part of my thighs. Is there something I can do to strengthen this area?*

What kind of pedals are you riding? Ones with too much float make the hamstrings and adductors work too much, which can cause premature cramping. I suggest limiting your float to the minimum your knees can handle (I use Speedplay Zeros). Too wide a seat or any bike-fit-related aspect could be an issue, as well. Additionally, you may want to emphasize movements which take place in the frontal plane—a neglected plane of motion for most triathletes and an obvious weak link in your development. Side lunges, especially coupled with upper-arm integration, would be a great place to start.

RUN-SPECIFIC QUESTIONS

- ***I seem to always get injured once I reach a certain level of running miles per week. Are there exercises I'm missing in my training routine which would make me more durable?***

Without knowing your training background and health history or analyzing your running form, it's easy to speculate but difficult to determine with 100% confidence the true etiology of your injury. In all likelihood, it's a combination of factors. Everyone has their individual threshold for miles over which the chances of injury increase exponentially. Maybe you've reached that level. Perhaps your run program is periodized incorrectly with intense sessions occurring prematurely or too frequently. How many days a week are you running? I'm a believer in frequency to build volume rather than duration of individual runs. Is your warm-up adequate? What about your cool-down and recovery strategies? Are diet and lifestyle sufficient to support your training endeavors? How's your cadence, your posture, your foot strike? The drills described in Chapter Four of Section Three will help anyone, regardless of level, to learn proper landing mechanics and improve ground-reaction time and proprioception. Just like dance or martial arts, running is a skill which can be broken down and practiced in pieces until it flows with unconscious competence. And, depending on where in your body you are consistently getting injured, I'd suggest incorporating the run-specific prehab exercises described in Chapter Five of Section Three.

- ***The run is my weakest discipline of the three. I focus on improving it with speed work and other quality sessions but was wondering if the weight room might be the missing piece.***

Strength training will make you more durable and give your legs the stiffness they need to effectively return energy to you with each stride. But you mention speed work, and I can't help but cringe a bit. Speed work is the icing on the cake, but most people don't have a cake yet. Strength needs to come before speed. So instead of repeats of 400s or 800s, I prefer to give my clients hill work which stimulates the aerobic/anaerobic system the same way. But because of the incline, the speed which must be run to elicit the same training response is less. Additionally, vertical displacement is decreased as the foot has less distance to fall before ground contact with the hill. Both of these factors equate to less impact forces while actually increasing the run-specific muscular stimulus of the workout. As for actual exercises I'd recommend, lunges, step ups, unilateral supine hip-extensions and unilateral squats would all be on the list. I'd also incorporate plyometric movements and running drills, too, of course.

• *I understand that improving cadence is one of the most efficient ways to run faster, but I seem to have trouble maintaining a quick turnover off the bike. Do you believe strength training can help?*

Yes, strength training can help. The drills, ladder work, and the explosive lower-body movements in Chapters Three and Four of Section Three will aid you in improving your ground-reaction time and turnover. The combination of heavy lift followed by explosive or quick movement helps train the body to react with speed and efficiency. Outside the gym, you need to program your neuromuscular system to run at a higher cadence (ninety and above) so that this rhythm becomes your default stride rate that you could run in your sleep. If your difficulty with turnover only manifests off the bike, you may want to look at your bike pacing (is it too fast for your fitness level?) or your bike cadence—pushing too big a gear on the bike can result in a slower run cadence as you "imprint" a slower rhythm into your legs right before the start of the run (not to mention tapping your limited glycogen supplies more than when using a higher cadence with less force per pedal stroke). Lastly, leg movement is predicated on arm movement. So concentrate on moving your arms faster and the legs will respond in kind.

261

• *I got outkicked for a place on the podium at my last race. Any suggestions for improving my final sprint?*

Trip the guy. No, seriously, tactical positioning may have been the issue as well as psychological state (which is related to fatigue which is related to training, nutritional, and health status). Gym work would again focus on the plyometric movements and the exercises from the PC phase of weights. This phase is, of course, built upon the two preceding phases, so proficiency in the AA and MS phases of training must be developed first. I'd also suggest incorporating what I call accels (also known as strides) into the majority of your runs, especially in the final miles of a long workout.

References

Anderson, T. "Biomechanics and running economy." *Sports Medicine*, 22 (2), 1996: 76-89.

Batmanghelidj, F. *Your Body's Many Cries for Water*. Falls Church, VA: Global Health Solution, 2008.

Bompa, T. "Periodization of Strength Part 3." http://www.ptonthenet.com/ articles/ Periodization-of-Strength-Part-3-Max-Strength-Phase-819.

Bompa, T. *Periodization: Theory and Methodology of Training*. Champaign, IL: Human Kinetics, 2009.

Bono, C.M. "Low-back pain in athletes." *Journal of Bone and Joint Surgery* (Am). 86-A(2), 2004: 382-396.

Brittenham, D., and G. Brittenham. *Stronger Abs and Back*. Champaign, IL: Human Kinetics, 1997.

Chek, P. *How to Eat, Move, and Be Healthy*. San Diego: Chek Institute, 2004.

Chek, P. *Movement that Matters*. San Diego: Chek Institute, 2000.

Chek, P. *Program Design*. San Diego: Chek Institute, 1995.

Chek, P. *Scientific Back Training*. San Diego: Chek Institute, 1995.

Chek, P. *Scientific Core Conditioning*. San Diego: Chek Institute, 1998.

Chek, P. *The Golf Biomechanic's Manual*. San Diego: Chek Institute, 2001.

Clark, Mike "Essentials of Integrated Strength Training: Integrated Neuromuscular Stabilization Training (Balance)." http://www.ptonthenet. com/ articles/Essentials-of-Integrated-Training.

27th Ed. Dorland's Illustrated Medical Dictionary. Philadelphia: W.B. Sauders, 1985. 900.

Fiebert, I.M. "An overview of functional progressions in the rehabilitation of low-back pain patients." *Journal of Back and Musculoskeletal Rehabilitation*. 3(4), 1993: 36-49.

Fowles, J., D. Sale, and J. MacDougall. "Reduced strength after passive stretch of the human plantar flexors." *Journal of Applied Physiology* 89, 2000: 1179-1188.

Hanna, T. *Bodies in Revolt.* New York: Holt, Rinehart and Winston, 1970.

Horning, A. "All Systems Clear." *American Fitness.* 1998.

Jemmett, R. *Spinal Stabilization: The New Science of Back Pain.* Orthopedic Physical Therapy Products, 2003.

Jones, N. *Human Muscle Power.* Champaign, IL:Human Kinetics,. 1986.

Kendall, F. and E. McCreary. *Muscles: Testing and Function with Posture and Pain.* Baltimore, MD: Lippincott Williams & Wilkins, 2005.

Kurz, T. *Stretching Scientifically: a Guide to Flexibility Training.* Island Pond, VT: Stadion Publishing, 2003.

Laughlin, T. "Total Immersion Handout." 2001.

Lewit, K. *Manipulative Therapy in Rehabilitation of the Locomotor System 3rd* Ed. Boston: Butterworth-Heineman, 1999.

Martin, D and Coe, P. *Training Distance Runners.* Champaign, IL: Human Kinetics, 1991.

Mattes, A. Isolated Stretching: *The Mattes Method.* Sarasota, FL: Aaron Mattes Therapy, 1995.

McClay, I and K. Manal. "Three-dimensional kinetic analysis of running: significance of secondary planes of motion." *Medicine and Science in Sports and Exercise* (11), 1999: 1629-37.

Nelson, Kokkonen, and Arnall. *Journal of Strength and Conditioning.* May 2005: 342.

O'Shea, P. *Quantum Strength and Power Training.* Patricks Books, 1998.

Poliquin, C. *The Poliquin Principles.* Chicago: Poliquin Performance Centers, 2006.

Reese, R. "Cycling and The Stick." 2002. http://www.thestick.co.nz/cycling.html.

Richardson, Jull, Hodges, and Hides. *Therapeutic Exercise for Spinal Segmental Stabilization in Low Back Pain.* New York: Churchill Livingstone, 1999.

Sapolsky, R. *Why Zebras Don't Get Ulcers.* New York: Holt, 2004.

Schlossler, E. *Fast Food Nation.* New York: Harper, 2005.

Schmidt, R and C. Wrisberg. *Motor Learning and Performance*. Champaign, IL: Human Kinetics, 2007.

Stitt, P. *Beating the Food Giants*. Manitowoc, WI: Natural Press, 1982.

Siff, M.C., and Y.V. Verkhoshansky. *Supertraining: Strength Training for Sporting Excellence*. Denver: Supertraining International, 2009.

Resources

www.chekconnect.com
www.chekinstitute.com
www.metabolictyping.com
www.powersystems.com
www.thestick.com
www.triumphtraining.com
www.westonaprice.org

Glossary of Terms

Amortization Phase—The time between the start of the eccentric movement and the start of the concentric movement.

Anabolic—The phase of metabolism in which simple substances are synthesized into the complex materials of living tissue. Associated with tissue repair and/or growth.

Axial Loading—Weighting of or the force applied to the axial skeleton.

Catabolic—The metabolic breakdown of complex molecules into simpler ones, often resulting in a release of energy. Associated with tissue destruction.

Closed Chain—Movements in which the force applied is not sufficient to overcome the resistance, so the body moves away from or toward the resistance.

Concentric Contraction—The term used for the development of tension in a muscle while it is being shortened.

Contact—In plyometric training, any time the foot touches the ground or landing surface.

Coronal Plane—Another term for Frontal Plane.

Cortisol—A glucocorticoid produced by the adrenal gland in response to stress; also referred to as hydrocortisone. This "stress hormone" is involved in the function of glucose metabolism, insulin release, as well as the immune system and inflammation response.

Cross-Crawl Pattern—Movements in which the arm and the opposite leg work together to stimulate biomotor integration.

Descents—In exercise, a step down in complexity or neurological demand.

DOMS—Delayed Onset Muscle Soreness. The term used to describe the pain and/or stiffness felt 24-72 hours after performing a movement which is new or different in intensity, volume, or frequency.

Dynamic Stability—The ability to maintain an optimal instantaneous axis of rotation in any joint(s) during movement.

Dynamic Stretching—Controlled, constant movement into and out of a stretch position to facilitate the range of motion without inhibiting muscular strength.

Eccentric Contraction—The term used for the development of tension in a muscle while it is being lengthened.

EPOC—Excess Post-Exercise Oxygen Consumption. The term used to denote the calories expended after cessation of exercise.

Equilibrium Reactions—Reflexes that work to maintain or regain control over the body's center of gravity so one does not fall; dominant when moving over a surface which moves underneath an individual.

Fascia— Layer of uninterrupted fibrous tissue that surrounds and penetrates muscles, organs, and other anatomical structures, effectively connecting the entire body.

Femoral Anteversion—A condition in which the femoral neck leans forward with respect to the rest of the femur.

Flicks—Quick, rhythmic movements of the arms and legs to restore non-physiological joint motion, relax muscles, and decompress joints so that the body may move without restriction.

267

Force Couple—Two or more muscles working synergistically to produce a particular movement.

Frontal Plane—A vertical plane which divides the body into front and back; movement occurs side to side.

Glucocorticoids—A class of steroid hormone predominately involved in carbohydrate metabolism.

Inner Unit—A term coined by Australian researchers Richardson, Jull, Hodges, and Hide, describing the functional synergy between the TVA and posterior fibers of the internal oblique, pelvic-floor muscles, multifidus and lumbar portions of the longisssimus and iliocostalis, and the diaphragm.

Inter-muscular Coordination—The interaction of two or more muscles during a muscular activity.

Intra-muscular Coordination—The interaction of individual muscle units within a muscle fiber.

Kinetic Chain—The term used to describe how the body functions as a system of chain links, whereby an action generated by or force acting on one part of the body affects the successive body part(s).

Kyphosis—An exaggerated outward rounding of the thoracic spine, specifically in excess of 35°.

Law of Facilitation—One of the neurological laws that states that when an impulse has passed once through a certain set of neurons to the exclusion of others, it will tend to take the same course on a future occasion; and each time it traverses the path, the resistance in the path will be smaller.

Lordosis—An inward curvature of the lumbar spine considered exaggerated if in excess of 35°.

Motor Program—A set of specific commands that are structured before a movement sequence begins.

Motor Unit—An alpha motor neuron and the muscle fibers it innervates.

Multifidus—One of the three types of muscles which make up the transversospinalis group. Spanning two to four vertebrae, they are part of the Inner Unit and play a key role in segmental spinal stabilization.

Neural Drive—A measure of the number and amplitude of nervous system impulses to a muscle.

Neurological Demand—The complexity of a specific action, generally increasing as the number of joints involved goes up and/or the platform off which the action is performed becomes less stable.

Neutralizers—Muscles which counteract unwanted and unnecessary movements of other muscles by producing an opposing action, thereby allowing for smooth, coordinated movements. See also *Synergists*.

Neutral Spine—The natural position of the spine, with the cervical, thoracic, and lumbar curvatures in good alignment, neither excessive nor deficient.

Non-dominant—Referring to the side of the body which possesses less motor skill than its corresponding counterpart.

One-Rep Max—The maximum amount of weight one can lift in a single repetition for a given exercise.

Open Chain—Movements in which the force applied is sufficient to overcome the resistance, so that the resistance moves away from or toward the body.

Parasympathetic Nervous System—One of the three branches of the Autonomic Nervous System (ANS), often referred to as the repair-and-rebuild or anabolic system. It is primarily responsible for digestion and elimination as well as stimulating the immune system.

Pattern Overload—Injury to soft tissues resulting from repetitive motion in one pattern of movement, or restricted movement in one or more planes of motion.

Pelvic Tilt—The anterior or posterior rotation of the pelvis. Ideal for a man is 4-7° anteriorly. Ideal for a woman is 7-10° anteriorly.

Phasic—Muscles composed of at least 51% fast-twitch muscle fibers. Primarily responsible for movement, and with an early susceptibility for fatigue, these muscles are prone to inhibition and react to faulty loading by weakening.

269

Prime Mover—The muscle primarily responsible for an action. Also called the agonist.

Pronation—A position of the foot (or forearm, when the radius crosses over the ulna to turn the palm down) combining dorsiflexion, calcaneal eversion, and internal rotation, which causes an inward rotation of the foot during heel strike and the subsequent ground contact during gait. It is the opposite of supination.

Prone—Position of the body when lying face down.

Reciprocal Inhibition—The simultaneous relaxation of one muscle encouraged by the contraction of its antagonist.

Righting Reactions—Reflexes that work to keep the head in a normal position, right the body to a normal position, and adjust the body in relation to the head and the head in relation to the body; dominant when moving over a surface which is stable or fixed.

Rotator Cuff—The name given to the supraspinatus, the infraspinatus, the teres minor, and the subscapularis which, working together, stabilize the glenohumeral joint.

Sagittal Plane—A vertical plane which divides the body into right and left halves; movement occurs forward and backwards.

SAID Principle—Specific Adaptation to Imposed Demands. A principle of training which dictates that the type of demand placed on the body controls the type of adaptation which will occur.

Stabilizers—Muscles which stabilize and/or support and protect a particular body segment while other muscles (prime movers) perform a movement.

Static Stability—The ability to hold the body in a particular position so that a task can be performed against any load placed on the body, including the weight of the body itself.

Static Stretching—A method of stretching involving an extended hold of a particular position for 30-60 seconds in an effort to lessen the sensitivity of tension receptors and allow the muscle to relax and elongate.

Stretch-Shortening Cycle—An eccentric contraction or lengthening of a muscle followed immediately by a concentric contraction or shortening of a muscle which, when sequenced appropriately, results in performance enhancement postulated to be a result of stored elastic energy.

Stretch Weakness—Weakness that results from muscles remaining in an elongated condition, however slight, beyond the neutral physiological rest position, but *not* beyond the normal range of muscle length.

Supercompensation—the period post-training during which, if training and rest parameters were both appropriate, the body responds to the stimulus by increasing its performance capacity.

Superset—Two exercises performed in a row before a rest interval is implemented.

Supination—A position of the foot (or the forearm, when the ulna and radius lie parallel to one another and the palm is facing up) combining plantar flexion, calcaneal inversion, and external rotation, which causes an outward rolling of the foot during the push-off phase of gait. It is the opposite of pronation.

Supine—Position of the body when lying face up.

Sympathetic Nervous System—One of the three branches of the Autonomic Nervous System (ANS), often referred to as the "fight or flight" nervous system. When activated, blood is shunted away from the organs of the body and to the working muscles in preparation for action, while the Parasympathetic Nervous System is proportionally inhibited.

Synergists—Muscles which assist the prime mover in acting on a joint. Often referred to as neutralizers, because they help control, or neutralize, extra motion from the agonists to make sure that the force generated works within the desired plane of motion.

Time Under Tension—The amount of time (per repetition) in which the muscle is under tension, measured as the sum of the eccentric, the concentric, and the time between the two phases.

Tonic—Muscles composed of at least 51% slow-twitch muscle fibers. Primarily responsible for posture with a late susceptibility for fatigue, these muscles are prone to hyperactivity/tonicity and react to faulty loading by shortening.

271

Transfer-of-Training Effect—In exercise, the more closely a particular movement resembles the activity trained for, the higher the likelihood of *usable* strength-transfer to that activity.

Transverse Plane—A horizontal axis which divides the body into top and bottom; movement occurring here is rotational.

Transversus Abdominus—(TVA) The deepest of the four abdominal muscles and part of what is termed the Inner Unit. This muscle provides the spine and pelvis the necessary stability without which the extremities could not fire effectively.

Upper Cross Syndrome—The term used to describe the muscular imbalance common among the active and sedentary alike, whereby the deep cervical flexors and scapular adductor muscles are weak and held in a lengthened position by facilitated pectorals, levator scapula, and upper trapezius—all of which tend to be short and tight. This results in a posture of excessive thoracic kyphosis and is related to a number of dysfunctions throughout the body.

Vertical Oscillation—In running, the amount of vertical displacement of the body which takes place with each stride.